Cambridge Studies in Biotechnology

Editors: Sir James Baddiley, N. H. Carey, J. F. Davidson, I. J. Higgins, W. G. Potter

4 Process development in antibiotic fermentations

T0245351

Process development in antibiotic fermentations

C.T.CALAM

Biology Department, Liverpool Polytechnic

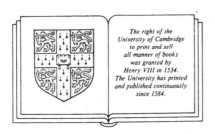

The right of the
University of Cambridge
to print and sell
all manner of books
was granted by
Henry VIII in 1534.
The University has printed
and published continuously
since 1584.

CAMBRIDGE UNIVERSITY PRESS

Cambridge

New York   New Rochelle   Melbourne   Sydney

CAMBRIDGE UNIVERSITY PRESS
Cambridge, New York, Melbourne, Madrid, Cape Town, Singapore, São Paulo

Cambridge University Press
The Edinburgh Building, Cambridge CB2 8RU, UK

Published in the United States of America by Cambridge University Press, New York

www.cambridge.org
Information on this title: www.cambridge.org/9780521304900

First published 1987
This digitally printed version 2008

A catalogue record for this publication is available from the British Library

Library of Congress Cataloguing in Publication data
Calam, C. T.
Process development in antibiotic fermentations.
(Cambridge studies in biotechnology; 4)
Bibliography
Includes index.
1. Antibiotics – synthesis. 2. Pharmaceutical microbiology
3. Fermentation. 4. Biochemical engineering. I. Title
II. Series
QR46.5.C35 1987   615'.329   86-26426

ISBN 978-0-521-30490-0 hardback
ISBN 978-0-521-06552-8 paperback

To teachers, colleagues, and friends in the field of industrial microbiology.

'We are coming into the region of guesswork,' said Dr. Mortimer. 'Say rather, into the region where we balance probabilities and choose the most likely. It is the scientific use of imagination, but we have always some material basis on which to start our speculations.'

A. Conan Doyle *The Hound of the Baskervilles*

Life can only be understood backwards, but it must be lived forwards.   Kierkegaard

Contents

Preface

Fermentation process development is a very wide field, and the variety of subjects and tasks involved, very great. One worker may be glad to have achieved 1 gram/litre of a new product, another, with an old one, is stuck at 30 g/l; yet others wrestle with poor or erratic growth, infections, or with economic problems. How can some sort of balance be struck when writing on such a subject? In the present case, an attempt has been made to present a simple account of the subject, illustrated by a few examples. The result is bound to be speculative and over-simplified, and the omission of so many valuable ideas must not be taken as a lack of respect for them. It is only possible to give a few pointers towards problems and to interesting areas of work, which may suggest further analysis of problems and ways to their solution and, hopefully, provide interest to those unfamiliar with the field.

I have to thank the late Professor J. S. Hough for suggesting the writing of the book, and my dear wife for her patience with the resulting decay of home and garden. I am also glad to acknowledge the help of firms and individuals in providing information: Dr J. P. Herman and Glaxo Research, ICI Plc, Agricultural and Pharmaceuticals Divisions, Dr S. W. Carleysmith and Beecham Pharmaceuticals, Dista Ltd, Liverpool, and Dyckerhoff AG, Gulheim, West Germany. I must also thank Dr I. S. Hunter for providing the stylised graph in Fig. 3.9d, and Dr Elizabeth Wellington for reading the drafts and making many helpful suggestions.

Part 1
Background

1   Introduction

1.1   Origins of the development of antibiotic processes

Dr Alexander Fleming first observed penicillin in 1928. A contaminant colony of *Penicillium notatum* growing on an agar plate covered with bacterial colonies had brought about the lysis of all the colonies around it. In further culture experiments, the disinfecting effect of penicillin was confirmed, but the techniques available at the time were insufficient to enable it to be extracted and tested further. Ten years later, Florey and Chain, with a large team of scientists at Oxford, managed to prepare extracts and demonstrate their efficacy. As a result of this, production began in order to supply the material to the armed forces, and the first use in the field began in 1943 in North Africa. In 1945–6, as supplies increased, penicillin became generally available.

Professor L. P. Garrod, a leading bacteriologist, commented later that no other such trivial observation as that of Fleming has had such momentous consequences. Fifteen years afterwards the mould was being cultivated on a gigantic scale to produce a substance of unexampled power. There was no other chemotherapeutic agent that could be used with such a complete disregard for possible harmful effects. Although its action is selective, it could be used to treat diseases that previously could only be dealt with with difficulty or not at all. Along with the sulphonamides, available in 1935, it dealt with half the emergencies occurring in medicine; it completely transformed the outlook, reducing fatalities to a minimum.

The production of penicillin involved major efforts in process development, and these provide a useful introduction to the present book.

In Britain, the immediate task was the production of material. Small surface-culture units were established for the purpose, and these were later expanded as agency factories on behalf of the government. Manufacture depended on the use of large numbers of milk bottles, handled using dairy machinery.

In America, where work began in 1942, bottle plants were established, but process development was concentrated on producing a practical manufacturing process using submerged culture. The main developments involved the following: improved media, especially media containing corn-steep liquor and lactose; the isolation of new strains and mutants that gave good results in submerged culture; and the development of

3

suitable laboratory and plant equipment. The amount of work done was enormous. Although stirred fermentations in pilot plant equipment were reported quite early (e.g. Stefaniak *et al.*, 1946), it was a considerable time before plant operations became really reliable. This was mainly because of the large amount of novel equipment that was required, and this could only be designed and modified in the light of experience. There were also the problems of infection. To some extent, the pilot fermenters give the impression of being crude. This was due to the practical talents of the Americans, who modified existing equipment to give a sturdy result. They also used standard parts, bought locally, so as to allow instant modification when necessary.

The isolation of the mutant Q176 (Johnson *et al.*, 1946) was a key factor. It made possible yields of 0.5–1.0 grams/litre (g/l), against previous yields of a few milligrams. Although large-scale production was in progress beforehand, manufacture reached a sound base in the early 1950s, with yields of 2–3 g/l by using new methods and mutants.

These developments were accompanied by the discovery of new antibiotics, for example streptomycin (1945), actinomycin (1946), chloromycetin (1947), terramycin (1949), erythromycin (1952), and cephalosporin (a new β-lactam) (1957). The semi-synthetic penicillins appeared in about 1956. As a result of these developments, the present enormous antibiotic industry has come into being.

The ability of the Americans to move so rapidly was, to some extent, due to their freedom of action as they entered the war, and also due to the availability of materials and capacity for plant construction. A main contributory factor was, however, the highly developed state of applied microbiology in the United States, through the influence of the solvents industry, the dairy industry, and other industries.

Some of the main needs for industrial progress became apparent from this early development work. It is convenient to summarise them here, as they provide the subjects to be expanded in the further chapters of this book. The requirements remain much the same, but the knowledge and experience that have been acquired since then have, of course, been greatly extended.

(a) Good production cultures, carefully selected for stability, and carefully preserved.

(b) A sound method for the production of the pre-production cultures used to start the main fermentation. This is an area where considerable skill is needed, and the expertise of those who work in this field is often overlooked.

(c) Well-designed and thoroughly reliable apparatus for stirred and shaken culture, able to operate continuously over long periods of time, indeed for many years, without breaking down.

(d) A carefully worked out support programme for batch operation.

Once, when a project student was in difficulty with a stirred
fermentation, it was suggested that he write down a list of all the
necessary preparatory steps, the completion of which was
necessary before the batch could be inoculated. He wrote down
22 items, mostly trivial, but all required for convenience and
success.
 (e) They say that a mother looking after children needs eyes in the
back of her head. This very much applies to development work,
where all sorts of things are happening, and it is easy to miss
significant items unless both eyes are open.
 (f) Good experimental records so that results can be recalled
whenever necessary.
 (g) A good knowledge of fermentation behaviour, held as a series of
mental pictures, which make it possible to quickly judge the state
and progress of a fermentation, and diagnose its state and future.
Suppose the pH is at 6.3 instead of 6.8. Is this because of (1) a
mistake in the medium and technique, (2) a hitch in the
proceedings, (3) infection, or because the pH meter is in error?
This is a simple case; there are many others that are necessary to
keep in one's head, as a doctor holds diagnostic signs.
 (h) A general background knowledge relating to fermentation work.
This enables scientific knowledge to be applied so that
experience of different antibiotic fermentations can be
correlated, and so that a basis is available for planning new
development work. This requires both information and
imagination.
 (i) The ability to combine current practical results with theory, so as
to identify the next steps in development, plan key experiments,
and also realise when new work of a particular kind is needed,
before such plans can be made.

1.2   The antibiotics as commercial products

The antibiotics belong to a group of substances referred to as secondary
metabolic products, i.e. substances that are produced by living organisms
and that appear to be unrelated to the main processes of growth and
reproduction. Secondary metabolic products are easily recognised in the
garden, where flowers, with their colours and perfumes, provide
immediate examples. Other secondary metabolic products of plants are
resins, essential oils, herbs, spices, and alkaloids, in which there is an
enormous trade. Animals also exhibit secondary metabolism in the
formation of colours and other substances. These natural products have
produced a vast and interesting literature.
Microorganisms, in turn, produce secondary metabolic products,

which appear as colours and odours, especially obvious in fungi and streptomycetes. These substances appear during growth and provide a means for the recognition and identification of species. Antibiotic activity is displayed by many microbes, and many of these activities have been identified and characterised. It is reckoned that some 7000 have been listed in the literature. According to Roberts (1984), world trade in antibiotics reached £5000 million in 1981, and this is still expanding. Of these antibiotics, the β-lactams (i.e. penicillin and cephalosporin C, and their derivatives) formed 65% of the whole. Other major antibiotics are the amino-glycosides, the macrolides (e.g. erythromycin), chloramphenicol, and the tetracyclines. There are also a number of other antibiotics sold commercially, including anti-tumour agents and fungicides, some of the latter being used in Japan to control diseases in rice. The plant growth hormone gibberellic acid may also be included.

The original work on antibiotics was aimed at their use in human diseases caused by bacteria. Interest has been extended to include substances that induce healing and the treatment of gastric ulcers. There is also interest in their possible use in plant diseases. Another important role is as models for new synthetic drugs. Many of the secondary metabolic products which have been described have a powerful physiological action, although they may not be suitable as drugs in their present chemical state. Because the identification of structures has now become much more rapid, such compounds could provide powerful leads towards new types of drugs for commercial development.

1.3   The nature of secondary metabolism

As noted above, the antibiotics belong to the class of substances referred to as secondary metabolic products, that is, substances that do not take part in the main life processes. Although these substances have been recognised for a long time, only recently has their role been recognised. It is now realised that they play an essential role in the ecological system, in recognition, attraction, and repulsion of other creatures.

The occurrence in microorganisms of complex, novel substances that are coloured or physiologically active led these also to be regarded as secondary metabolic products. On the whole, these substances have been regarded as arising by chance, perhaps as a result of the shunting of surplus intermediates into metabolic sidelines. It is unlikely, however, that the complex systems of enzymes required for this purpose would occur without purpose. Demain (1983) comments on the secondary metabolic products as antagonistic agents, symbiotic agents, sexual hormones, effectors of sporulation and germination, metal transporters, etc. that offer the producing organism an opportunity to survive in the competitive arena of nature. Their relation to differentiation is also stressed, as has been deduced by workers such as Bu'Lock *et al.* (1974) and Chater & Merrick (1976).

The biosynthetic routes to many antibiotics are well known. The starting points are mainly amino acids (e.g. in making penicillin) and acetyl-CoA (in making tetracyclines and other polyketides), with isoprene and shikimic acid also being involved. Antibiotic production commences at some point in differentiation, often during sporulation, with quantities of the starting materials being diverted for the purpose. Process development consists essentially of modifying the metabolic system so that diversion of material and biosynthesis are greatly increased. The problem is to modify the mechanism of growth so that a hyperactive system of secondary metabolism can operate successfully, without damaging the growth system that supports it. This requires the availability of robust mutants and well-balanced conditions of growth that can work efficiently for as long as possible.

1.4   Stages in development

It is possible to distinguish several stages in development work. These will be discussed later, but it is convenient to mention them briefly here and establish some sort of nomenclature for strains at different levels of productivity. This classification is summarised in Table 1.1.

The initial step, involving minimal work, is intended to aid in the experimental testing work in which the antibiotic's future is determined. There is an advance to a high yield as early manufacture begins. The later development stages are likely to take a considerable time and may result in very high-yielding processes. It should be said, however, that the development to very high and maximum levels of yields often depends on improvements to the fermentation system, so that the production time may well be doubled. This means that the productivity of the cells per gram is not increased as fast as is necessary at first.

It should be stressed that the increases and times required are purely notional. In any given case, the values may vary considerably. Some processes may achieve, say, 7 g/l only after very many years, and during development there may be periods when no advance is made. With some specialised products, sold in small amounts, lower yields may be quite acceptable.

1.5   The literature of process development work

Defining the literature of development presents a problem because development is about the future, while the literature is about the past. For this reason it is best to consider the subject as a series of ideas concerned with development that grow out of present and past experience and point

Table 1.1. *Advances in yield during process development*

Step	Class	Yield range (g/l)	Notional yield (g/l)	Advance	Time (years)
0	Wild strain	0.05–0.2	0.1	—	—
1	Medium yield	0.2–1.0	0.5	×5	0.5–1
2	High yield[a]	2.5–7	4	×8	3–6
3	Very high yield	8–15	10	×2.5	5–10
4	Maximum yield, super, mutants	30–100	35	×3.5	10–20

[a]I.e., high yield relative to wild strain.

the way to the future. The identification of these ideas and their expansion is, of course, a matter of opinion, and there is a very open field for action. Meetings and conferences are often the best source of information and ideas.

In writing of these subjects here, it is not possible to go into very much detail. It is also assumed that in the well-written areas of biochemistry and microbiology the reader will be able to turn to a textbook to fill out the brief sketches that are given here.

At the present time a number of books are appearing that are of great interest in development work. Some of these are listed in the bibliography. To obtain a view of the field, it is valuable to look through the volumes of *Biotechnology and Bioengineering*, as these contain a great range of information of different degrees of comprehensibility. References are also given in the following text, which, it is hoped, will provide further references to the many ideas that are involved in process development work.

2 The microorganisms and methods of culture

Before we move to a detailed account of the behaviour of antibiotic fermentations and their development, the present chapter is intended to briefly describe the organisms used, methods of culture, mode of growth, and general behaviour, based on a consideration of ordinary microorganisms rather than special high-yielding mutants. This will be illustrated by two student-type experiments. However good the descriptions may be, they can never be as useful as a visit to a laboratory where work is in progress, which will bring out the methods used and the type of expertise required for success.

2.1 The isolation of antibiotic-producing microorganisms

2.1.1 General screening techniques

Antibiotic-producing organisms are obtained as a result of search programmes. Fungi and streptomycetes are isolated from soils and other materials by plating samples and picking off suitable colonies. This procedure is outlined later in this chapter. The isolated colonies are transferred to slopes and tested in a suitable manner. A modern isolation and test system has been described by Nolan (1986). Targets of 10 000–100 000 colonies, tested annually, are achieved by growing the isolates in small cups in a stationary block, using a liquid medium. The solutions obtained are then diluted and screened *en masse*, the tests being conducted in similar blocks. These are then read using a computerised system that not only records the test results but also compares these results with those from previous tests (held in memory) and with a target pattern and picks out any that show the desired pattern. This avoids a personal and painstaking study of the data, which can be time consuming and subject to error. Such a system may produce 20–100 new isolates that fulfil the initial criteria for suitability. About 10% of these may pass the initial stage of the subsequent testing stages.

The screening programme may involve up to ten tests judged suitable for the purpose. Bacteria, mutated bacteria, or enzyme systems that are considered to represent the desired target effect may be used in these tests. The substances sought may be antibacterials, but at present the substances include many other targets, illustrated, for instance, by the recent discovery of asperlicin, a non-peptide antagonist of

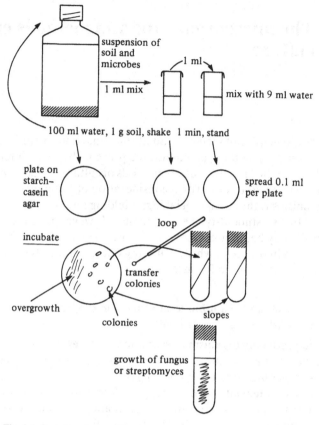

Fig. 2.1. Isolation from soil.

cholecystokinin, a hormone governing many bodily activities (Chang *et al.*, 1985).

2.1.2 Example – isolation of streptomycetes from soil, and test for production of antibiotics

This example illustrates some of the methods used in this field of microbiology.

One gram of soil is shaken with 100 ml of sterile water for 1 min to bring into suspension spores of microorganisms or fragments of hyphae. After allowing the suspension to stand, to allow the soil to settle, a 1 ml sample is added to 9 ml of water in a test-tube or vial, and the dilution is repeated 2–4 times. Samples of 0.1 ml are then transferred to agar plates containing a suitable medium, such as starch–casein agar. Four to five plates are used for each dilution. The suspensions are then spread over the surface of the plates, using a bent glass rod which is sterilised by dipping it in alcohol and igniting to cause flaming. The plates are then incubated for 5–7 days at 25 °C. The general scheme is illustrated in Fig. 2.1.

On examination of the plates it will be found that some are completely overgrown, while others show small colonies of streptomycetes. Plates showing 20–30 colonies should be selected. The colonies resemble small mould colonies, having a whitish background, with the central area coloured grey, brown, pink, or other colours. The strong smell of the streptomycetes will be noted.

It is best to test several soils at once, as the ease of observing and separating the streptomycete colonies depends on the other inhabitants of the soil. Often mould colonies will be seen, and plates may be covered by slimy bacteria. It is common to add small quantities of antibiotics to the agar (e.g. 1 unit/ml) to reduce the invading microbes.

Colonies may be tested for antibiotic activity by removing small pieces of agar that bear colonies, and placing them on nutrient agar plates seeded with *Staphylococcus aureus*. After 24 h incubation, the bacteria grow, and clear zones of activity will be seen around some of the colonies. Unfortunately, this activity is not usually due to antibiotics of any importance. If desired, the streptomycetes may be transferred to slopes and cultured for further examination. Starch–casein medium has the following composition (g/l): starch, 10; casein, 0.3; KNO_3, 2; NaCl, 2; $MgSO_4 \cdot 7H_2O$, 0.05; $CaCO_3$, 0.02; $FeSO_4 \cdot 7H_2O$, 0.01; agar, 13. The pH is 7.0–7.2.

2.2   The main types of antibiotic-producing microorganisms

The main types of microorganisms used for antibiotic production are the fungi and the streptomycetes, although many other types produce secondary metabolic products of different kinds. The relationship between the fungi and the streptomycetes is summarised in Table 2.1, which indicates the main features of each group.

The eukaryotes and the prokaryotes are sharply divided. The eukaryotes (which include the plants and animals) have a complex nucleus that is enclosed in an envelope and has at least several chromosomes. The cells are relatively complex, for instance the respiratory and energy-forming systems are enclosed in the mitochondria. In the prokaryotes all these aspects appear to be simplified, but actually the metabolic system is equally structured by other means. One of the main differences is size, the fungal threads being much larger than in the streptomycetes. As will be seen, the wall components and the storage products are also different. Bacteria, consisting of rods and cocci, are included for comparison with the streptomycetes, being very similar in composition.

Table 2.1 mentions a few genera typifying the different groups. These are only a few of the very many and varied genera and species that exist in each group, and they have a very wide range of morphological and other features. Over 600 species of *Streptomyces* are described in the literature.

Table 2.1. *Types of microorganisms concerned with industrial antibiotic production*

Division	Group	Characteristics	Width (µm)	Cell walls	Storage products	Nucleus	Important genera
Eukaryotes	Fungi	thread-forming; aerobic; aerial spores; haploid or diploid	2–5	cellulose; chitin	polysaccharides; fats	enclosed; several chromosomes	*Penicillium*; *Cephalosporium*; *Fusarium*
Prokaryotes	Actinomycetes	thread-forming; aerobic; aerial spores	0.2–0.6	murein; techoic acid	polyhydroxy-butyrate	unenclosed; single chromosome; plasmids	*Streptomyces*; *Nocardia*; *Streptoverticillium*
	Bacteria	unicells, rods, or spheres; aerobic or facultative anaerobes	1–2	murein; techoic acid	polyhydroxy-butyrate	unenclosed; single chromosome; plasmids	*Bacillus*; *Pseudomonas*

The fungi range from the simple monocellular yeasts through to the mushrooms and toadstools.

An important difference between fungi and the streptomycetes is that the latter are sensitive to antibiotics, including their own, because they are, in effect, gram-positive bacteria.

Microbial cultures, such as those used for antibiotic production, are referred to by genus and species, for example *Penicillium chrysogenum*. The actual cultures used for experimental work may be isolates from soil or mutants of them, and they are referred to as strains, though the term 'mutant' is often used. Mutants and strains are usually given a reference number. For example, the original oxytetracycline producer, *Streptomyces rimosus*, has the number NRRL 2234, this being the catalogue number at the Northern Regional Research Laboratory, where it was deposited.

In spite of the differences between fungi and streptomycetes, it is convenient to consider them together, since from a practical point of view they have so much in common.

The identification of isolates and their careful preservation are important parts of isolation and selection work.

2.3   General description of the microorganisms

The chemical composition of typical dry cells is, approximately, 40% carbon, 10% nitrogen, 1% sulphur, and 10% ash (mostly sodium and potassium salts), with the remainder being oxygen (about 40%). The analysis can also be considered in terms of carbohydrates and protein. The results obtained depend on the species, the medium used for growth, and the age of the culture, but they may average 10–25% carbohydrate and 30–60% protein.

Microbial cells consist of a strong cell wall composed of fibrils of polymeric materials and lined with a cytoplasmic membrane that seals the cell and controls its input–output activities. In fungi the fibrils are composed of cellulose and chitin, while in prokaryotes the components are polymers of amino sugars and amino acids and the techoic acids, consisting of poly-alcohol phosphates. The outer layer of the wall is often rich in polysaccharides which form a mucilaginous layer, often seen in scanning microscope photographs.

Within the cell wall, the essential mechanisms of the cells are contained within the liquid cytoplasm. These are, essentially, the enzymes and the nucleus, which controls the operation of the cell. The enzymes may be in solution, but many key groups of them are attached to the cytoplasmic membrane or to other membranes within the cell or are located in groups on protein particles. In the fungi, the energy-producing system is situated within the mitochondrion. In the prokaryotic streptomycetes the nucleus consists of a single chromosome, which lies free within the cytoplasm. In the fungi, the nucleus possesses several chromosomes, which are enclosed in an envelope. These cytological details are too extensive and complex to describe further here, and the reader should refer to a textbook to obtain a fuller account.

The hyphae of fungi and streptomycetes are not sub-divided by cross-walls, though in fungi compartmentalisation is visible, as at intervals partial cross-walls appear. These cross-walls have a central pore, which is plugged if autolysis occurs so as to seal off the dying area. The absence of cross-walls means that the cytoplasm is continuous along the hyphae, so that particles of material that are required for extension can be passed forward over a considerable distance to the growing tip.

Both streptomycetes and fungi show obvious life cycles. On agar media, after initial growth and formation of mycelium, conidiophores develop, from which spores (i.e. conidia) develop in chains or in masses. In the fungi, spores may be round or oval, and quite small, or they may be large and complex in form. In streptomycetes, tubular conidiophores develop that are straight, wavy or spiral, and these break up into chains of spores, which may be smooth or rough, and white or brown-blue or other colours.

The different kinds of fungi and streptomycetes show common patterns of behaviour, but there are many individual differences in behaviour between strains, and it is necessary to treat each case on its merits.

2.4   Media and culture conditions

2.4.1   Media

Microorganisms are grown on liquid or solid media containing the nutrients necessary for growth. These nutrients supply carbon, nitrogen, sulphur as the main cell constituents, together with inorganic substances and precursors or growth factors in small amounts. Of these, phosphate acts as a buffer, but it is also an important cell constituent, acting as a carrier of energy and in other ways. Calcium carbonate is frequently added to neutralise acidity, but it also has a physical effect on the form of growth. Media are solidified with agar.

Table 2.2 gives a list of some of the substances used in media. In the case of automatic pH control, ammonia is frequently used as an alkali, thus making up the nitrogen used for growth. Fungi and streptomycetes will grow at pH levels as low as 5.0, but the optimum working range is usually 6.5–7.0. At pH values above 7.5–8.0, free ammonia appears in the medium and is toxic. The preferred temperature is usually in the range 24–28 °C.

It is common practice, with antibiotic production, to use complex nutrient sources. These are at least partly insoluble. They are broken

Table 2.2. *Materials used in fermentation media*

Ingredients	Types of material used
Carbon sources	carbohydrates: sucrose, molasses, glucose, lactose, maize meal, starch, liquefied starch vegetable oils: arachis (peanut) oil, maize oil, sunflower oil, etc.
Nitrogen sources	inorganic: ammonium salts, ammonia, sodium nitrate, urea organic: corn-steep liquor, soya meal, ground peanuts, cotton-seed meal, fish meal, etc.
Inorganic salts	major components: potassium phosphate, sodium sulphate, calcium carbonate trace elements: Mg, Fe, Zn, Cu, Mn, Mo, Co
Vitamins	yeast extract or individual substances
Precursors	as required in each case
pH control	buffers: phosphate, calcium carbonate direct control with alkali

down by enzymes given off by the cells (diastases, proteases) at a slow and steady rate that is well adapted for the controlled growth of the cells and production of antibiotics. If starch is used, it might produce a very thick and viscous medium, so a heat-resistant *Bacillus licheniformis* diastase may be used to liquefy the solution.

Two of these natural products which are frequently mentioned are corn-steep liquor and cotton-seed meal. Corn-steep liquor (CSL) is a by-product of the corn-starch industry and contains a mixture of lactic acid and peptides, plus inorganic salts. It is supplied as a thick liquid containing 50% solids, pH 4.0. Cotton-seed meal is sold under the names Pharmamedia and Proflo, by Traders Protein, Buckeye Cellulose Corporation, Memphis, Tennessee 38114, USA. It contains 60% protein, 20% carbohydrate, 6% fat, plus salts and fibre. According to Queener & Swartz (1979), modern corn-steep liquor is less effective than the older type, and cotton-seed meal is preferable for penicillin production. Soya meal is also commonly used. It contains 55% protein, and is largely soluble in water. These proteins can be obtained from millers and from health shops.

There is naturally a reluctance among inexperienced workers to use these natural products. In fact, they represent animal and human foodstuffs, which are prepared to consistent standards. Although they may interfere with cell estimations, they provide many operational advantages and economies.

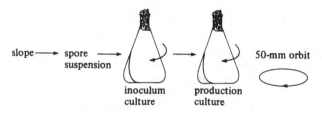

slope ⟶ spore ⟶   ⟶   50-mm orbit
suspension

inoculum   production
culture   culture

Fig. 2.2. Shaken culture method.

Trace elements may be provided by the use of a concentrated solution, for example by adding 20 ml/l of a solution of (g/l): $MgSO_4 \cdot 7H_2O$, 2.5; $FeSO_4 \cdot 7H_2O$, 0.6; $MnSO_4 \cdot 4H_2O$, 0.2; $CuSO_4 \cdot 5H_2O$, 0.2. Similar small amounts of zinc, cobalt, or molybdenum may be added, but detailed requirements may have to be studied.

Although the fungi and streptomycetes grow well on many media, there are usually strong interactions between the medium and antibiotic production, requiring a special investigation to give optimal results.

2.4.2   *Methods of culture: example of shaken culture*

Fungi and streptomycetes grow on solid media in the form of colonies of mycelium covered with spores. These colonies can often be seen on moist bread or other foods that are left around in a cupboard or other suitable place. Microorganisms can also grow on stationary liquid medium; a felt of mycelium develops on the surface. This method was originally used for penicillin production. The technique is not as easy as it looks, as the mycelium is apt to grow only around the edge, or partially submerged in the medium, and the method has other disadvantages. Microorganisms are grown industrially in stirred and aerated conditions, with the cells totally submerged in the medium. The necessary agitation and aeration is provided by shaking the flasks, or by the use of a jar fermenter, with a stirrer and inlet pipe for the air. Shaken and stirred fermentations are provided with temperature control, and precautions are taken to avoid infection by other organisms.

The general methods employed are conveniently illustrated by describing the production of oxytetracycline (OTC) in shaken culture. The process is illustrated in Fig. 2.2.

The medium is prepared using liquefied starch, corn-steep liquor, soya flour, ammonium sulphate, and calcium carbonate. The medium (35 ml) is distributed into 250-ml Erlenmeyer flasks, and 0.5 ml of sunflower oil is added. The flasks are plugged with cotton wool and sterilised by steam pressure in an autoclave, so as to heat the flasks to 120 °C for 20 min. This requires 1 bar pressure. After cooling, a slope is used to inoculate some flasks, which are incubated on the shaker at 25 °C, at 250 rpm with orbits of 5 cm. As soon as a thick culture has been obtained (36–48 h), the production flasks are inoculated with 3 ml of culture and incubated on the shaker. The thickness of the inoculum can be judged by pouring a little culture into a sample tube, and standing it for 10 min, when it should be seen to be 75% full of cells. The production stage, with a good mutant, takes 4–5 days. The oxytetracycline is insoluble in water, so the culture must be acidified and shaken for 5 min before filtration. The solution can be tested for oxytetracycline by the ferric chloride method, or by the cylinder and plate method, using *S. aureus* as test organism. Descriptions of these methods will be found in the literature.

2.4.3 Culture preservation

In process development work, the careful labelling and preservation of master cultures is essential to success. The master cultures are specially prepared and set aside to ensure that workers can always go back to the original strain and find it in excellent condition. It must always be possible to obtain a desired strain, in good condition, whenever required, after an interval of a few months or many years.

Several methods of culture storage can be used.

(a) Slopes may be held at 4 °C for up to a few weeks.

(b) Streptomycetes are often stored as slopes at −70 °C, and they will keep for several years. Spore suspensions can be held in the same way, in 20% glycerol.

(c) Spore suspensions of streptomycetes or fungi, in sterile skim milk solution (5 g/l) may be added to good-quality, powdered, activated silica gel (5 ml in test-tubes, sterilised at 150 °C), cooled in ice, and well mixed. The plugged tubes are kept in sealed jars at 4 °C, and remain good for several years.

(d) Master cultures of fungi and streptomycetes are frequently stored in liquid nitrogen, using specially designed containers. The spore suspensions (in water or 20% glycerol), sealed in 1-ml ampoules, are cooled slowly and immersed in the liquid nitrogen in easily removable racks.

(e) The preferred method of storage is to freeze-dry spore suspensions in serum or other suitable liquids, in small amounts in 1-ml ampoules. The liquid is frozen and the ampoules attached to a vacuum drying apparatus. When the pellets are dry, the ampoules are sealed *in vacuo*. These will keep for many years. Special apparatus designed for the purpose is usually used (Edwards High Vacuum, Crawley, W. Sussex).

Details of the methods described will be found in the literature. It should be said that culture preservation and management requires technical skill and organisational expertise, and most large firms have a special department for this purpose.

2.4.4   Culture rundown

Streptomycetes and fungi are both subject to an effect referred to as rundown. This is a form of nuclear instability that causes strains to show morphological variations and also loss of productivity. Quite large differences occur between strains in this respect, but it is safer to expect rundown than otherwise. Rundown should be prevented by careful preservation and storage. Here, much seems to depend on the skill and experience of the workers concerned, some being more successful than others, but it is always possible that rundown will occur after long-term storage.

This effect has long been known to bacteriologists, since pathogenic bacteria lose toxicity and infectivity on storage in the laboratory.

One reason for rundown is the occurrence of natural variation, whereby, on growth, small numbers of low-yielding variants appear. On sub-culture these may outgrow the parental strain, so that productivity is lost. In such cases, the original strain can be recovered by plating, though, from experience, this may require a good deal of effort. On the other hand, in many cases the capacity for high yields is lost and cannot be recovered by selection, though, in some cases mutation and selection may provide a partial solution. The reason for this serious and irreversible rundown is not known.

When rundown occurs, there are nearly always morphological changes. During the process of change, it may show as small sectors of a different colour, or mosaic effects may be seen if the surface of colonies are examined under a strong hand lens. Specks may be seen on the reverse. Experts nearly always make a careful study of production cultures, with a lens, before further investigations. It is important that all cultures are well described, so that even slight changes can be observed at a later date.

2.5   Identification of the microorganisms

The methods used will be described briefly, but it will be realised that experience is needed to achieve success, mainly because the morphological details are not always clear to beginners though they are obvious enough when once experienced. Fungi are usually identified as far as genus, the identification of species being more difficult. Streptomycetes are usually identified as far as species, of which there are very many.

There is a particular difficulty with fungi. These may be considered in two groupings, haploid or diploid. In nature, fungi often exist as diploids, i.e. two haploid forms (not necessarily identical) that conjugate to produce an elaborate form of growth with specialised spore-bearing systems. An example is the major group of ascomycetes, in which the spores are produced in small sacs, many of which are enclosed in larger vessels, among the hyphae. These are often seen on decaying wood. Their identification is a special subject in itself. *Penicillium chrysogenum* is haploid, being a partner in the diploid *Eurotium*, and the asci can appear in some forms of the *Penicillium* genus. The majority of the fungi used commercially are haploids, which multiply and sporulate without conjugation, and are referred to as Fungi Imperfecti. These produce spores in different ways, are coloured, and are identified by different means.

The Fungi Imperfecti are divided into two groups, with light or dark spores. Among these, identification is by the nature of the structure of the spore-bearing apparatus, by the shape and size of the spores, by the presence or absence of cross-walls in the spores and by other means. The colours of the colonies are also used as features for identification.

The genus *Streptomyces* consists of thread-forming gram-positive bacteria. The species are identified by the colour of the spore mass, as seen on colonies on agar, by the smoothness or roughness of the spores, and by whether the spore chains are straight, wavy (flexuous), or spiral. They are further subdivided by their ability to grow on a series of ten sugars. There are a large number of species and many of them are poorly differentiated by these tests. This method was devised by Pridham & Tresner (1974) and is given in *Bergey's Manual of Determinative Bacteriology* (1974), and it is probable that modifications will be proposed in future editions. Recently, Williams *et al.* (1983*a,b*) have reclassified the *Streptomyces* species in 60 clusters and developed a computer identification system using 41 tests. No doubt further developments of this approach will continue.

In work in the field of antibiotic production, careful descriptions of the strains being used are essential, and identification of cultures is also important. This is to make sure that changes that could cause loss of productivity do not occur. Especially when a large number of cultures are in use, this can give rise to difficulty, especially when programmes continue for several years.

In production work, mutants and selected cultures are nearly always used. Although these retain the main features of the parental strains, they can differ in many details, apart from increased productivity. Here again, appearances and important features must be carefully recorded.

2.6   The genetics of fungi and the streptomycetes

Because of their eukaryotic and prokaryotic nature, the genetics of the fungi and the streptomycetes are essentially different. With the fungi, only the imperfect state will be considered. In any case, only an outline of the subject will be attempted (as it affects process development work) and the subject will be referred to again in Chapter 9. The whole subject of microbial genetics is too large and important, and expanding too rapidly, to attempt any kind of summary.

In the Fungi Imperfecti the nucleus contains a small group of chromosomes, each containing a DNA chain that is coded with genetic information. During growth the nucleus duplicates without undergoing the complex processes associated with the perfect state. Gene modifications can be brought about by mutation or by recombination.

The method of recombination commonly used was devised by Pontecorvo, Roper & Forbes (1953), by means of the so-called parasexual process. For this purpose two complementary, biochemically deficient mutants are grown together. As the two kinds of hyphae develop, cross-linkages occur through which the nuclei migrate. A state is reached (heterokaryosis) in which the two types of nuclei are together in the cells. Such hyphae can grow slowly on minimal medium, mature, and sporulate. Since each spore contains a single nucleus, the different parent strains are recovered. During growth, however, a small number of diploidisations occur, some between unlike haploid nuclei. Spores containing such nuclei have twice the normal volume, due to their diploidy. They will grow on minimal medium. The diploids break down, directly or after mutation, to give recombinants with nuclei containing parts of both of the parental nuclei. Both the parental nuclei and the recombinants may be haploid or diploid. Some of these recombinants give high yields. The main advantage is that they bring new genetic material to high-yielding strains which may have lost vigour or be difficult to use in different ways.

In the case of the streptomycetes, the nucleus consists of a single strand of DNA carrying the genes. The strand is usually represented as a circle, starting from the point of replication. Very extensive mapping of the streptomycetes has been carried out, and very much information of their behaviour has been accumulated. Increases in productivity can be obtained by mutation and by recombination in much the same way as with the fungi. In the case of recombination, the position is complex, since apart from the differing responses of different strains there is also the intervention of fertility plasmids, common in many bacteria. If serious work is to be attempted in recombination, a careful study of this subject is desirable, starting from work in Professor Hopwood's laboratory in the early seventies (cf. Hopwood & Wright, 1976). More recently, extensive work on gene insertion, using plasmids, has been carried out with the streptomycetes, allowing very detailed studies of *Streptomyces* genetics and the production of new strains. Unfortunately, owing to the complexity of the enzyme systems involved in antibiotic production, this is not as yet a suitable means for directed methods.

With both fungi and streptomycetes, the use of protoplasts is of great

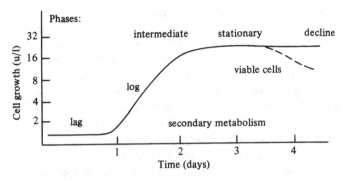

Fig. 2.3. Cell growth pattern. u/l, Units/litre.

advantage for the insertion of genetic material into cells and for recombination. This involves the enzymic removal of the cell wall, giving cells bounded only by the cytoplasmic membrane. When the resulting protoplasts are mixed, under the right conditions, new forms can be grown up, showing extensive genetic recombinations (Peberdy, 1979; Ball, 1983; see also Demain & Solomon, 1986, pp. 154–215).

2.7 Microbial cell growth

2.7.1 The growth curve

When inoculated into medium, under good conditions and free from restrictions, bacteria grow according to a well-recognised pattern, passing through a series of well-marked stages. The resulting curve is shown in Fig. 2.3. This pattern, or one similar to it, also occurs with fungi and streptomycetes, though production curves are usually managed to give a modified pattern, intended to give maximum production.

The initial phase is referred to as the lag phase, during which the cells may have to change from the resting to the growth condition. This may require from 12 to 24 h, or longer. In industrial work the lag is avoided by inoculating with actively growing cells. In the next phase rapid growth commences, the cell concentration doubling over a certain period known as the doubling time. This may range from 0.3 to 5 h, or more, depending on culture and conditions. If the logarithm of the cell concentration is plotted against time, as has been done in Fig. 2.3, a straight line is obtained, hence the name used.

Three full doublings are shown. Since logarithmic growth implies a steady conversion of materials to cells, cell activity can be regarded as in a balanced state. The log phase may continue for 1–3 days. At the end of this time, whether because the nutrients are exhausted, or because the oxygen supply becomes inadequate, or because toxic products are formed, growth slows down (intermediate phase) and then ceases (stationary phase). During the latter phase, the cells tend to die off, so that in bacterial cultures the viable count falls below the total count.

If secondary metabolism occurs, it is usually expected to start at the end of the log phase or during the intermediate or stationary phase, being induced as unbalanced growth commences in the so-called idio-phase. Thus the loss of balance is regarded as a trigger for secondary metabolism. The idio-phase has thus come to be regarded as essential for secondary metabolism, the unbalanced metabolism providing excesses of intermediates, which are used for the production of the new products. With mutants this pattern does not always hold, production starting during the balanced log phase and continuing during the stationary phase.

Fig. 2.3 shows a series of transitions as growth passes from one phase to the next. It is interesting that these events occur with bacteria. They presumably arise because of exhaustion of a particular nutrient and adaptation to another, with slowing at the end due to the presence of staling factors. With fungi and streptomycetes, the cells show morphological changes, with the culture thickening and then thinning, thus adding a number of variable factors to the system.

2.7.2   *Morphological changes during growth*

The thread-forming microorganisms extend by elongation at the tip. The number of growing points is thus relatively low, compared with bacteria where each cell can extend separately. None the less, thread-formers can grow exponentially. This is because the cells or compartments in the hyphae all produce particles of cell-wall materials, which then migrate to the growing tip and are inserted into the extending thread. Since a long section of the thread is involved, there is plenty of material for growth. If the production of particles is high, they may accumulate at points in the hypha, and from these points branches may arise. The form of development of the hyphae and the production of sporophores and spores are controlled genetically, in response to conditions. A detailed model of this process has been developed by Prosser & Trinci (1979).

Growth on the surface of solid on stationary liquid media

When spores of streptomycetes or fungi are grown on solid media, the spores germinate after 12–24 h, and germ tubes emerge. From these a radially growing system of hyphae develop, forming mycelium. After a few days, a new stage develops, with the formation of colours and odours, and this results in the appearance of spores. The colonies are circular, white at the edge with a central coloured and sporulating area, and have a diameter of 0.5–2 cm. The colonies may be flat, domed, or wrinkled. After a time the colonies begin to decay, and there are changes in appearance and colour.

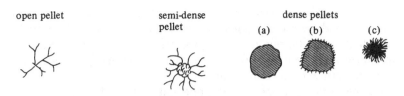

Fig. 2.4. Types of pellets in submerged culture.

A similar form of growth occurs on stationary liquid media. Here, the colonies form a confluent mat, with the lower part immersed in the medium. With surface culture, the culture is clearly not uniform, there being both submerged and aerial mycelium. This presents a difficulty in the understanding of microbial behaviour; this difficulty is avoided in submerged culture.

Growth in submerged culture
Cultures may be started from spores or from pre-grown, young mycelium. The inoculum is added to the culture medium and grown on a shaker or in a stirred fermenter.

As with surface cultures, growth starts with the production of hyphae. These, however, grow out in all directions instead of only in a horizontal plane. Growth may occur as individual hyphae, which grow and branch, or in small masses of hyphae, which grow in the form of complex pellets. As a matter of convenience, all individual particles of hyphae or mycelium are referred to as pellets. In a few cases, the culture may grow as single cells, referred to as 'yeast forms', in both laboratory and production cultures, but this is uncommon.

Most commonly, growth takes place as more or less complex pellets. These occur in different forms, and during a fermentation, they may undergo a series of changes. They represent a complex pattern of morphological and biochemical behaviour. Various types of pellets may be produced, which will be discussed later, but it is convenient to describe them briefly as belonging to three main classes (see Fig. 2.4), based on microscopic appearance.

Open pellets, often small (0.1–0.5 mm diameter), consist of growing, branching hyphae that radiate from a point, there being no central mass of mycelium. Semi-dense pellets show a central dark mass, from which emerge hyphae that grow well and may be branched (1–3 mm diameter). Dense pellets (0.5–5 mm diameter) vary considerably in texture and appearance. Typical examples are shown: (a) consists of hyphae fused together, often autolysed; (b) is a similar mass of material but with a thin layer of short hyphae on the outside; (c) consists of a mass of thickened hyphae radiating from a central point, with the outer tips in a healthy condition. Pellets vary very much in appearance and condition, and these are mentioned as typical of common types referred to in the literature. Individual fermentations are often associated with particular types of mycelial growth, and the correct shape and form of the pellets is a marker of correct fermentation behaviour.

Starting from spores, the pellets appear after 36–48 h, earlier if a mycelial inoculum is used. In complex media containing solids like calcium carbonate, there is a tendency to form small open pellets; in synthetic media denser pellets are obtained. The type of pellets formed depends on many factors. Fungal pellets are larger and often complex, while streptomycetes tend to form very tiny pellets with a relatively simple structure. As growth occurs, dense pellets tend to become larger, but open pellets remain the same size but become more numerous. For given conditions, behaviour is regular, and the state of a fermentation at any time can often be judged by the appearance of the pellets.

The biochemical state of the mycelium is reflected in the pellets. When different conditions for growth are used and the pellets change in size and shape, the corresponding changes in metabolism reflect these biochemical changes, as well as any effects pellet morphology may have on gas transfer and mixing. These aspects are further discussed in Chapter 5.

The shape of the pellets has a number of effects on the fermentation. Small, soft, open pellets give a sludgy form of growth that restricts oxygen transfer, while small, dense, sandy pellets give a lower viscosity and better transfer of oxygen to the medium. Large pellets may restrict oxygen distribution within the pellets, causing inefficient metabolism. There is thus an optimal form of pellet for each fermentation.

If the reader has difficulty in visualising a submerged culture, an idea can be obtained by adding 40–50 g of pin-head-sized, ground oatmeal to 500 ml water, and stirring with a spoon. A large number of particles are seen, which sink rapidly, after the manner of small dense pellets. If the mixture is heated, with stirring, just to boiling, and then cooled, the liquid is now full of pale grey, slightly viscous material, which, on pouring, shows a grainy effect. This resembles the appearance of many fermentations with the open type of pellets, except that the coloration and odour are lacking. The thick suspension of the swollen oatmeal gives an impression of the difficulty likely to be experienced in securing efficient stirring and aeration.

3   Microbial Physiology

3.1   Introduction

Microbial physiology is the study of the manner in which cells grow and live. It is concerned with their metabolism, growth, reproduction, and response to the environment. In the case of the production of antibiotics, the formation of these substances must be added to these functions. The environment becomes that of submerged fermentation systems, which are affected by the physical conditions used and the effect that the presence of the organism has upon these physical conditions.

Chapter 2 gives a general account of the behaviour of the streptomyces and fungi. In the present chapter a more-detailed account of the behaviour of antibiotic-producing strains is given. The subject is a large one, and it is only possible to give those aspects which are of practical interest. The discussion will also be based on the behaviour of relatively high-yielding strains, stressing features of this behaviour that are important in commercial production of antibiotics and that can be used as a basis for a consideration of advanced development work.

The chemical and biological behaviour of the microorganisms is very complex, involving many reactions, within and without the cells. To attempt to describe such a multi-dimensional system is almost impossible. Workers in the field, therefore, adopt the physiologist's view and consider the cell as a mechanism through which material flows, giving rise to cells and products. The interaction between these flows, the properties of the cells, the conditions used, and the regulatory systems involved can then be considered in terms of systems engineering, without going into too much detail about the biochemical and other mechanisms involved, so as to produce a relatively simple model. Because each microorganism is unique, it is hard to lay down any sort of average or normal behaviour that could be used as a basis for all fermentations, but it is possible to start with a simplified model that can be gradually extended to meet individual situations.

The main components in the cell system are the consumption of nutrients and oxygen, and their conversion to growth, along with the production of carbon dioxide and antibiotics. Throughout process development work, these activities, and the way they are related and regulated, and the way they interact with the conditions in the fermenter form the basis on which further development proceeds. Regulation is an

25

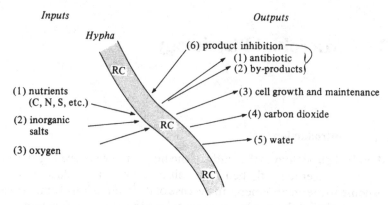

Fig. 3.1. Material conversions in antibiotic production. RC, respiratory centres.

important aspect of the equation, as its modification is a main factor on which increased production of antibiotics depends.

The complexity of the subject has been mentioned. The question arises as to whether it is necessary to take such a difficult approach to process development. Why not side-step theory and work entirely by trial and error and intuition? It is true that during the early stages this is just what is done. Medium variations and mutations are carried out, usually with useful results. Later, however, conditions become more restricted as the effectiveness of the culture system reaches its limits, and a deeper understanding becomes necessary so as to be able to ask the right questions and seek answers to them. Novel ideas and suggestions should never be neglected, as they are often useful and lead to progress. In the end, more than empiricism is needed to find the best way forward.

In describing and discussing the physiology of antibiotic production, the various aspects of the subject will be illustrated by examples from two differing fermentations, the production of penicillin and of oxytetracycline.

3.2   The cell as a production mechanism

It is convenient to begin with a general consideration of the growth and production system and to bring out some of its main points before going into detail. As already indicated, antibiotic production occurs as an offshoot of the main metabolic pathways, and it is possible to present a general concept of the cell's main activities as a simple flow or conversion pattern. A scheme of this sort is presented in Fig. 3.1, which indicates the main inputs and outputs involved.

The scheme in Fig. 3.1 has been reduced to a minimum, for the sake of clarity. These inputs are shown, (1) a main source of organic substances,

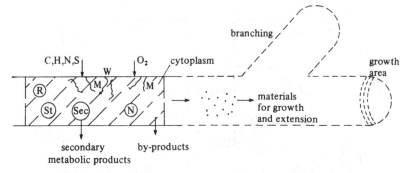

Fig. 3.2. Cell physiology and biochemistry of a cell compartment in a growing hypha (main areas of metabolism). W, wall; M, membrane; N, nucleus; R, ribosome; St, storage products.

supplying carbon and nitrogen, (2) an inorganic source comprising phosphate, magnesium, and trace elements, and also sulphate, and (3) oxygen, which is converted to water in the respiratory centres, while intermediate materials are also used, producing carbon dioxide. This is represented in the hypha by RC, indicating the respiratory centres.

The ratios for the conversion of nutrients (mainly carbohydrate) to the first three output components, antibiotic, by-products, and cells, is readily appreciated, as all contain about 40% carbon. The direct conversion of carbohydrate to 10 g of antibiotic and 40 g of cells would require 50–60 g of carbohydrate for synthesis, but the requirement of energy would roughly double this amount. This is a subject that will be discussed later. Cells contain about 10% ash, mainly sodium, potassium, phosphate, and magnesium. Growth could be limited by any of these components, including inorganic materials.

In Fig. 3.1, a loop indicates an important factor in the situation, (6) product inhibition. This refers to the fact that the fermentation may be stopped by the toxicity of the antibiotic or the inhibitory effect of some of the by-products. For this reason high-yielding strains must be highly resistant. It is considered (Martin *et al.*, 1979) that the extent of production is equal to the resistance of the cells to the products. Thus, although this is not part of the material flow, it must be considered alongside it.

Some further aspects of cell physiology are shown in Fig. 3.2. The diagram shows a section of a growing hypha, with a growth area near the tip. The main features of a single compartment in the hypha are shown, comparable with the reactions shown in Fig. 3.1. As previously described, the compartment is separated from the medium by a strong wall and the cytoplasmic membrane. The cytoplasmic membrane is semi-permeable and is selective in allowing the entry and exit of nutrients and products.

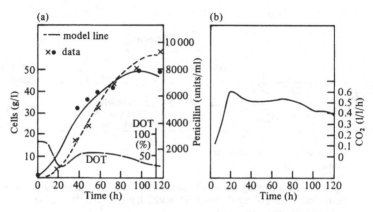

Fig. 3.3. Fermentation data: penicillin, Run 30. (a) Growth and production; (b) CO_2 output rate. DOT, dissolved oxygen tension.

This process is enzymically controlled, and could have been included as a feature of Fig. 3.1. The cytoplasm consists mainly of water, which has enzymes, storage particles and small molecules of sugars, amino acids, and other substances involved in metabolism suspended or dissolved in it. These materials are referred to as the cell pool. Many of the main enzyme groups, such as the tricarboxylic cycle, are arranged in special arrays; in prokaryotes they are on membranes or attached to the wall, and in eukaryotes they are in the mitochondria. The cytoplasm also contains the nucleus. Thus the cell, with its elaborate (if microscopic) structure, its external enzymes which dissolve its nutrients, and its toxins that inhibit other organisms, is a highly organised structure, and not just a 'bag of enzymes' as used to be said.

Fig. 3.2 shows a single centre of secondary metabolic activity. There is no evidence that all secondary activities depend on such a single location, but it is often found that when this activity begins in microorganisms, several types of product appear at about the same time, suggesting a degree of co-ordination.

Having thus outlined the conversions taking place during a typical fermentation, the next stage is to consider these processes of growth, respiration, and antibiotic production in more detail, considering the system as a group of material flows, organised by the cell mechanism. This will be done by considering an experimental fermentation.

3.3   Illustrative example: the penicillin fermentation
3.3.1   Fermentation data

It is convenient to discuss the main biosynthetic areas, growth, production, and respiration in a practical way, so the various

Table 3.1. *Terms used in discussing fermentation results*

General
Concentration of cells, g/l = x; age = T(hours (h))
Rate of growth, g/l/h = dx/dt
Specific rate of growth, $(dx/dt)/x = \mu$
The corresponding values and symbols for antibiotic production are:
  p (units (u)/ml or mg/ml), dp/dt, Q_p
For oxygen consumption, dO_2/dt, Q_{O_2}, etc.
Yield of cells: per gram sugar, Y_G; per litre O_2, Y_{O_2}
DOT = dissolved oxygen tension, as % of saturation
Respiratory Quotient (RQ) = $(dCO_2/dt)/(dO_2/dt)$
Oxygen transfer coefficient, K_{La}, see Section 3.3.7

Components: materials involved in medium, etc.

Factors: physical conditions, temperature, etc.

Parameters: ratios between reactants, e.g. Y_{CO_2}, m, and p in Equation 3.1

relationships will be considered in relation to a penicillin production batch, i.e. Run 30, described by Calam & Ismail (1980), the results of which are summarised in Fig. 3.3. In considering these material flows, concentrations are given as grams/litre (g/l), and flows are given as g/l/h, or as specific rates (g or units(u)/g cells/h). Some of the main expressions used are given in Table 3.1. It is usual to work in g/l, rather than in molecular values, for the sake of simplicity, especially as cells have no definable molecular weight.

The penicillin batch in Fig. 3.3 (Run 30), carried out in a 5-l fermenter, using a lactose + corn-steep medium, with a feed from 60 h, gave rapid growth which slowed down after 48 h. Penicillin production began at about 12 h and continued to 120 h. Dissolved oxygen fell at 24 h, then rose to 50% of saturation, subsequently slowly declining. The other graphs give the rate of output of carbon dioxide, and the rates of growth (dx/dt and μ) and of penicillin production (dp/dt and Q_p). Although the fermentation conditions were relatively crude, the results were typical for penicillin batches of this type, and they will be discussed in more detail later.

3.3.2 Terms used

Table 3.1 summarises some of the main terms used in discussing these subjects.

3.3.3 Carbon balance in Run 30

The conversions shown in Fig. 3.1 suggest that it should be possible to obtain a balance between carbon consumed and carbon in the products

Table 3.2. *Penicillin batch, carbon balance*

Inputs per litre	g/l	%C	C (g/l)	Outputs per litre	g/l	%C	(g/l)
Lactose	41	42	17.2	Cells	50.5	43[a]	21.6
Corn-steep liquor	37	35	13	CO_2	58 litres	27	29.0
Arachis oil	20	85	17	Penicillin	6	50	3.0
Sucrose	30	42	12.6	Soluble			
Precursor	2.5	66	1.3	residue[a]	31[a]	43[a]	13.5
Inoculum[b]	10	43	4.3				
Total			65.4	Total			67.1

[a] Based on McCann & Calam (1972).
[b] Includes dissolved material.

for a batch like Run 30. From the reference it was possible to prepare such a balance. Taking into account the necessary approximations, the results (Table 3.2) were quite good. There was a fair spread of carbon in the medium ingredients, while the bulk of the output carbon was in the cells and carbon dioxide. Allowance was made for the soluble residue in the medium, such as occurs with this fermentation. Only a small amount of carbon went to the product.

Although the carbon balance came out quite well, it involves some uncertainties. In spite of this, it is of use in checking experimental work. If unaccountable errors occur, it means that some reaction that has not been allowed for is involved, or that there has been an error in technique, which must be cleared up.

Balancing can be carried out at any stage of a fermentation. Balancing can also be used to measure growth, or carbon dioxide production, provided all the other values are accurately known. These estimations are by difference and therefore include all the error values. Unless the whole situation is quite clear, these indirect measurements carry a degree of risk.

It will be seen from Table 3.2 that nearly half the carbon input was converted to carbon dioxide, i.e. it underwent combustion for the formation of energy. The conservation of energy in microorganisms is good, about 40% being converted to ATP. The remainder is lost as heat. This is of practical importance, as the heat raises the temperature of the fermenter. The input of power by the stirrer also contributes heat. This heating is important technically because it requires cooling. In a large fermenter, several tonnes of carbon may be combusted during a batch, producing a great deal of heat. Cooling is likely to be difficult if ample cold water is not available.

3.3.4 Relation between respiration, growth, and production

A special feature of microbes is their rapid rate of growth; doubling times are in hours, rather than in days or weeks as with plants. Therefore all cell processes also proceed at a rapid rate. Physiologically, respiration occupies a prominent place in this process. It involves two main activities, the transfer of phosphate ions (i.e. ADP $\rightleftharpoons$ ATP) and a corresponding redistribution of hydrogen atoms, and the decomposition of carbon compounds (via glycolysis and the tricarboxylic acid (TCA) cycle) in the cell. Although, in the microorganisms, this may occur with or without the involvement of oxygen, antibiotic-producing strains are normally strictly aerobic. The pattern of these conversions determines the respiratory quotient (RQ), i.e. the ratio of carbon dioxide produced/oxygen consumed. The RQ therefore indicates the type of conversion taking place. It is usually 1.0 when sugar is being converted to CO_2, and 0.6–0.7 when fatty acid or alcohol is the substrate, but it may fall as low as 0.3 when partly oxidised products are being accumulated, as can occur in a number of cases in antibiotic fermentations.

Since respiration is so prominent, and because all cell activities require energy, it may be assumed that some quantitative link should exist between the amounts of oxygen consumed and carbon dioxide formed, and the quantity of cells produced. Since the RQ can vary, the consumption of oxygen should be a better measure, but if, as in the case of the penicillin fermentation, the RQ is usually high and steady, it is reasonable to use CO_2 data as a basis. The value found by us is 0.95, however the value has to be checked in case it varies, which it might well do with some media and conditions. Experimentally CO_2 is easier to measure than oxygen, if only one of the two is being measured.

With antibiotic fermentations, it will be recognised that the main uses of energy will be (1) cell production (2) cell maintenance, and (3) antibiotic production and other secondary metabolism. This can be expressed by the equation (per litre of oxygen):

$$\frac{dx}{dt} \cdot \frac{1}{Y} + m.x + p = \frac{dCO_2}{dt} = -\frac{dO_2}{dt} \cdot RQ \tag{3.1}$$

where Y is the yield of cells produced or consumed, m is the maintenance coefficient (Righelato *et al.*, 1968), and p is an allowance for antibiotic production. It has been found (Ryu & Hospodka, 1980) that 1 g of penicillin requires 2.2 l of oxygen.

This equation is used here mainly in connection with the penicillin fermentation, and it is assumed, for simplicity, that RQ has a value of 1.0. This is reasonable with penicillin, but with other fermentations the situation would have to be carefully checked, as mentioned above. Carbon dioxide is convenient for the indirect estimation of cells, as it is a

32   *Microbial physiology*

pure substance and easily measured. The indirect measurement of cells is a subject often discussed, and different methods are preferred by different workers, many preferring the method of carbon balancing.

It will be seen that Equation 3.1 is useful because it brings together all the processes in the fermentation. Fig. 3.3b gives the carbon dioxide output rates for Run 30 (Calam & Ismail, 1980), and Fig. 3.3a shows calculated values and found values for growth. Good fits were obtained using the parameters $Y = 2.6, m = 0.0075, p = 0.07$. These values differ from those originally preferred by Calam & Ismail (1980), as they give a better fit at the end of the fermentation. It will be noticed that the data point at 24 h is well above the calculated curve. This is due to the presence, in the complex medium used, of a quantity of insoluble organic matter, which dissolved during the subsequent 24 h. This batch was chosen as an example to illustrate this aspect which is a common problem in development work.

Equation 3.1 is used here as a general relationship, which will be referred to at a number of points in the book to illustrate different aspects of fermentation behaviour. The values given for Y, m, and p vary with the medium, the strain, and the conditions. Values obtained by Righelato *et al.* (1968) were $Y = 2.08, m = 0.017$. The value of m tends to be higher with synthetic media.

3.3.5   *Sugar consumption and growth*

Pirt & Righelato (1967) compared sugar consumption against cell growth, using the equation:

$$\frac{-\,ds}{dt} = k \cdot \left(\frac{dx}{dt}\right) + m \cdot x \tag{3.2}$$

with values in grams. The amount of sugar used for penicillin production is small, and is combined with the maintenance requirement.

To check the relationship, the figures calculated for a penicillin batch in a 30-l fermenter were used, as given by Calam & Russell (1973). A good fit was obtained, as shown in Fig. 3.4, with the values $k = 0.7, m = 0.02$. Values obtained by Pirt & Righelato were $k = 0.5, m = 0.02$.

3.3.6   *The relation between growth and antibiotic production*

It was recognised early that optimal production was associated with a particular pattern of growth. Reviewing a number of microbial fermentations giving different products, Gaden (1959) concluded that with antibiotics, production was usually maximal subsequent to the peak rates of growth and sugar consumption and was not directly linked to the growth rate; there were some fermentations where this link seemed to be closer, such as in the production of oxytetracycline. Later, Shu (1961) developed a simple enzyme-decay model to explain the dynamics of

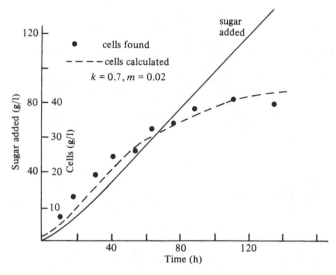

Fig. 3.4. Sugar consumption and growth, based on Run 4 (Calam & Russell, 1973).

product formation. He applied this successfully to several fermentations, including penicillin. This equation was later used by Calam & Ismail (1980) to relate production to growth. After a careful investigation of penicillin fermentations in continuous culture, Pirt & Righelato (1967) concluded that there was a relation between production and growth rate, which could be summarised by concluding that the productivity (Q_p) was constant above a critical value of 0.012 g/g/h; below this value, Q_p fell away rapidly. This view has been influential in the discussion of fermentation optimisation by several experienced workers (Ryu & Humphrey, 1973; Queener & Swartz, 1979). By the application of this rule, it is possible to optimise the length of a fermentation. There have been suggestions in recent papers, however, that production can continue beyond this rate of growth. For a recent review, see Hersbach, Van der Beck & Van dijck (1984).

A view of the position with Run 30, based on data from Fig. 3.3, is given in Fig. 3.5, which shows rates and specific rates of production and growth, and a graph of Q_p in terms of μ. The maximum rate of production (dp/dt) occurred in the middle of the fermentation (40–60 h), Q_p being highest at about 24 h, during initial growth, and then falling, but the increase in cell concentration maintained dp/dt for a considerable time. Eventually production tails off, Q_p falling sharply at low values of μ. This type of production curve is typical of fermentation processes at this stage of development. Later, the persistence of production, even at zero growth

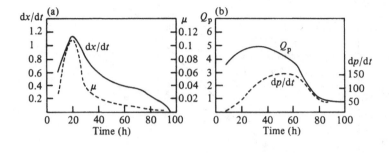

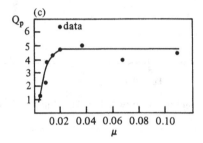

Fig. 3.5. Growth and production rates, Run 30. (a) Growth rates; (b) production rates; (c) specific rates.

rate, will be discussed further, and other aspects of the subject emerge in the example of the oxytetracycline fermentation at the end of this chapter, such as the effect of inhibitors that can arise in the fermentation itself.

From the point of view of process development, it is of practical importance to establish a link between growth and production, as a means of finding clues to optimisation. The view taken here is that at some fairly early stage of the fermentation (e.g. from 12 h to 3 days), with different processes and high-yielding mutants, secondary metabolism is triggered by one of the steps of differentiation (Bu'Lock *et al.*, 1974) and then continues as long as conditions within the cell remain favourable. Taking Run 30 as an example, penicillin production was triggered after about 12 h and, from Fig. 3.3, continued for 4–5 days. Since the cells are growing during this time, this process must include the fact that some are becoming active, while some are losing their activity, there being a changing concentration of cells during the fermentation period. These concentrations can be estimated graphically fairly simply, by drawing on a piece of graph paper: (1) the original growth curve, (2) the same curve set back 12 h, i.e. when the cells become active, and (3) the same curve set back further, corresponding to the age at which the cells become inactive.

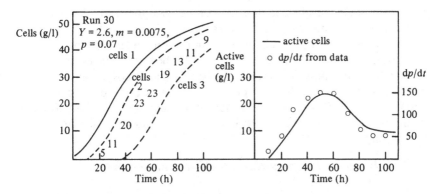

Fig. 3.6. Calculation of active cells and production rate.

The location of the third curve is judged by trial and error. The differences between curves (2) and (3) then give the concentrations of active cells. On multiplying this value by the maximum value of Q_p (Fig. 3.5), the production rates (dp/dt) for the batch can be obtained, and the production curve can be calculated. This procedure is shown in Fig. 3.6. The agreement is obviously satisfactory.

It will be noted from Fig. 3.6 that the third curve is set back 30 h from the second one, i.e. that the cells have an active life of only 30 h. This span varies considerably. For example, with Run 9 (Calam & Ismail, 1980), with synthetic medium, the span of activity was 90 h, suggesting a much more stable production system. This view was supported by the fact that at one point the sugar feed system broke down for 12 h, with production continuing after its restoration without substantial change.

In this chapter on cell physiology, sections 3.3.4, 3.3.5, and 3.3.6 are all concerned with the complex interactions between the processes of growth, respiration, and antibiotic production. The example of Run 30 is useful for this purpose. The result was good for a fermentation of this kind, dating technologically some 25 years ago. The data concerning the interacting factors was limited, as often the case in development work. Equation 3.1 gives a useful, if approximate, means of co-ordinating growth, respiration, and production; the relation between growth and production is also shown in Figs. 3.5 and 3.6. As has been said before, the fermentation system involves growth, and the appearance and then the disappearance of biosynthetic activity. Although the details are limited, this co-ordination of cell activity is well brought out. Here, the active span of the cells is relatively short, and penicillin production only lasted about 80 h. This emphasises the disadvantage of this relatively undeveloped process; much effort is involved in producing a mass of cells, but they are only used effectively for a limited time. To improve the position, the production stage must be extended 2–3 times, so as to exploit the possibilities of the process. This defines the work to be done in the later stages of development, especially in maximisation, and aspects of the work to be done will be introduced shortly. In the earlier stages of development, it is possible to work empirically and discover ways to increase production. As the work proceeds, it is more and more necessary to understand the fermentation as a mechanism that can be quantified and manipulated on the basis of its working processes and their quantitative relationships.

3.3.7   Oxygen transfer requirements: effect of stirring and cell concentration

In this discussion, oxygen concentration and oxygen transfer rates will be referred to as ml/l and ml/l/h, at 20 °C.

As shown in the previous section, an ample supply of oxygen is needed to produce and sustain a high concentration of cells in an efficient state. Oxygen supply to the culture is needed, both because of the amount required for growth, etc., and also to allow an adequate concentration of oxygen in the medium, generally reckoned to be in the range of 1.5–2.5 ml/l (25–40% of saturation; i.e. 5.5 ml O_2/l at 25 °C and 1 bar pressure of air). The transfer of oxygen and the concentration in solution depends on the mechanical ability of the fermenter to transfer oxygen to the culture. The culture must be managed in such a way that its demand for oxygen (ml/l/h) is not excessive. This means that the rate of metabolism of the culture and the degree of stirring and aeration must be matched.

The oxygen transfer rate to a fermenter is given by the equation:

$$\text{Oxygen transfer rate (OTR)} = K_{La}(C_I - C_L) \qquad (3.3)$$

where K_{La} is the transfer coefficient (in h^{-1}), C_I is the concentration of oxygen in the medium, in contact with the gas phase, when saturated, and C_L is the concentration at a particular time.

In a typical case, the percentage of CO_2 in the effluent gas was 0.70%, with an RQ of 0.95, and an airflow rate of 1 l/l/min. This corresponds to an oxygen transfer rate of $7.0 \times 60/0.95$, or 442 ml O_2/l/h. The dissolved oxygen meter read 55% saturation, or $5.5 \times 0.55 = 3.0$ ml/l. From the equation,

$$422 = K_{La}(5.5 - 3.0)$$
$$K_{La} = 442/2.5 = 177 \ h^{-1}$$

with 38 g/l cells in the culture.

It is possible to measure the oxygen transfer capacity of a fermenter by filling it with a solution of M/20 sodium sulphite and M/200 copper sulphate, and stirring and aerating and measuring the residual sodium sulphite, iodimetrically, every few minutes. With the fermenter used in the present instance, total conversion to sulphate required about 15 min. Calculation of the oxygen utilisation rate, with the oxygen concentration at zero, gave a value for K_{La} of $720\,h^{-1}$, corresponding to an oxygen uptake rate of $3.2\,g\,O_2/l/h$. Large fermenters are usually designed to give at least $4\,g/l/h$ (Imperial Chemical Industries Ltd, 1975).

It is evident that the presence of cells considerably reduces the rate of oxygen transfer. The effect depends on the thickness and viscosity of the culture, and the type of pellets produced. The degree of interference therefore depends on the particular strain used and the type of medium.

The example quoted was based on a fermenter 15 cm diameter, with a stirrer 10 cm diameter at 660 rpm. Using a complex medium, it was capable of producing penicillin with a good degree of efficiency, but a prolonged fermentation with continued production was not possible because a heavy growth of cells reduced oxygen transfer too badly. The fermenter could thus be regarded as having a limited biological space (Hockenhull & McKenzie, 1968). This limitation presents a general problem in process development work, which has to be taken into account in the planning of fermentation research.

3.3.8   The formation of by-products

Fig. 3.1 indicates that by-products may be formed alongside the main antibiotic during the fermentation. By-products may be of various kinds.

(a) Primary products such as gluconic or succinic acids, produced due to distorted metabolism.

(b) Secondary metabolic products which may be modifications of the main product, more or less closely related to it. These include, for instance, the various streptomycins and rifamycins, or the anthracyclines formed alongside the tetracyclines. Rhodes, Booth & Somerfield (1961) have described a number of benzophenones that occur in the griseofulvin fermentation, some being precursors of the main product.

(c) Other secondary metabolic products, such as geosmin and methyl-isoborneol, which give the characteristic odour to the streptomycetes.

(d) Unidentified substances, for example the increased level of dissolved matter that occurs late in the penicillin fermentation (McCann & Calam, 1972) to the extent of 10–15 g/l.

(e) Residual materials from the medium, these substances being used or only partially digested by the microorganism.

The presence of complex by-products in the filtered culture can interfere with the extraction and purification processes. Provided they are non-toxic and present in small amounts, these substances may have little effect on the fermentation itself. If large amounts are produced, they can

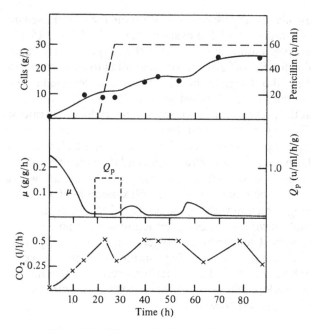

Fig. 3.7. Penicillin: metabolism of wild strain.

be harmful since they reduce the amount of material available for production, and, if acidic, they can upset pH control. If by-product formation requires oxygen, it can reduce the amount of oxygen for the production of the desired product.

During fermentation research it is easy to overlook the formation of by-products. They should be given consideration, however, as they can give rise to several undesirable effects, for example the waste of nutrients caused by their synthesis, interference with extraction and purification, and limitation of production due to product inhibition, all of which are harmful to progress.

3.3.9   Penicillin production by a wild strain

As a contrast to the results just described, obtained with the mutant DC2/14, a batch was run in a 40-l fermenter using a wild strain isolated from an old culture of NRRL 1951, which the wild strain closely resembled. The conditions used were the same as those described by McCann & Calam (1972). Under these conditions, DC2/14 behaved much as it did in Run 30. The results with the wild strain are shown in Fig. 3.7. Further details have been given by Calam (1982). The fungus grew in the form of large, very dense, orange pellets, with a slightly rough surface, in contrast to the smaller and looser pellets produced by DC2/14. The growth curve showed a series of separate phases, similar to those described by Duckworth & Harris (1949) with the mutant Q176. These phases of growth were reflected in the curve for the production of carbon dioxide, which showed troughs corresponding to each phase. Penicillin production began at the end of the first growth phase, lasted about 12 h, and did not recur. Old reports, with early mutants, also showed an early peak to production, in 66–72 h (Stefaniak *et al.*, 1946). Thus the impression given is that while mutants can give a smooth pattern of growth and production, in the wild strain the various processes are much more sharply defined and separated.

3.4   Growth and differentiation

Although varying patterns of growth have been described, for example germination, branching, and the formation of pellets, the impression has been given that this growth occurs smoothly, though growth may be disturbed by lack of oxygen or nutrients in the medium. In fact, the growth of microbes, as in plants, proceeds through a series of steps, each giving rise to its own form of growth as the organism develops. This sequence of steps is referred to as the process of differentiation. Based on the behaviour of higher organisms, it can be understood that as each differentiation step is completed a signal is given that starts the next step. The signal usually implies the disappearance of the substance holding the current step, and the appearance of a new signal for the next one. A number of regulator substances are known in plants.

The account given here will be based on the streptomycetes. The fungi, which has a considerable literature, probably behave in a rather similar manner. One important subject of study is *Dictyostelium*, which is described in the textbooks. The micro-cycle described by Smith & Galbraith (1971) is also of interest in this connection.

A practical problem in antibiotic research is that cultures are usually conducted in submerged culture, so that the changes observed in surface culture do not appear. Many improved mutants also change their pattern of growth, suggesting changes in differentiation in submerged culture. In submerged culture, however, there are frequently changes in the mode of growth, such as fragmentation of pellets, which probably reflect differentiation effects, and which are usually referred to as transitions. They are frequently associated with changes in metabolism.

Transitions and differentiation are important factors in process development and will be frequently referred to in later chapters. It is not an easy subject to understand, and individual readers will have to form their own views on the subject.

Recalling previous comments, the induction of secondary metabolism is seen here as a step in the pattern of differentiation. This relationship is

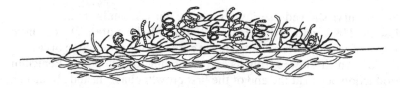

Fig. 3.8. Development of streptomycete colony (stylised).

illustrated by the following examples: the development of spore coloration in *S. coelicolor* (Chater & Merrick, 1976); a type of chemical differentiation (Bu'Lock *et al.*, 1974) shown by the formation of a series of substances by *Gibberella fujikuroi*; the appearance of an antibiotic in the first step towards the formation of spores in *Bacillus subtilis* (Mandelstam, 1969).

3.4.1   The process of differentiation

When strains of the streptomycetes are sown on to agar, the spores germinate and form hyphae that grow below the surface of the agar. These form a stiff waxy layer that rises above the surface of the agar (Fig. 3.8). From this layer arise fine aerial hyphae, among which develop another type of hyphae, often apparently stiff and shiny. Some of these are shown in Fig. 3.8. They are commonly hooked or develop into spirals. They develop cross-walls, giving small compartments within which the spores develop. Finally, the sheath, i.e. the outer wall of the conidiophore, collapses around the spores and may leave a rough or smooth surface. The conidiophores and spore chains may be straight, wavy, or in spirals. The spores may be white or may be grey, brown, red, blue, or other colours.

As described, the process involves six developmental steps: (1) germination, (2) formation of substrate mycelium, (3) formation of aerial hyphae, (4) production of conidiophores, (5) formation of the spore chains, (6) formation of secondary metabolic products (colours, odours, and antibiotic). It is evident that each of these stages will involve at least several differentiation steps.

The process of sporulation in *Streptomyces coelicolor* has been studied by Chater & Merrick (1976). Thirteen steps have been recognised in differentiation, commencing with the signal to start the reproduction phase, and ending with the final synthesis of the spore wall and the development of the grey colour. Many of the genes involved have been mapped. Some of the processes involved, such as the formation of septa and the walls of the spores, have been studied in detail. This differentiation behaviour has some resemblances to that observed in *Bacillus subtilis*.

3.4.2   Bio-regulators

An important development in the understanding of differentiation occurred about 20 years ago, when Professor A. S. Khokhlov, Academy of Sciences, Moscow, isolated from *Streptomyces griseus* a substance, referred to as A-factor, that restored sporulation and streptomycin production to mutants that had lost these functions. In fact the apparent double deficiency was really due to the loss of the ability to produce A-factor. Reviewing the situation recently, Khokhlov (1982) drew attention to three types of factors affecting differentiation. These included sex factors, such as trisporic acid, certain antibiotics, and the bio-regulators (or autoregulators) such as A-factor and related substances. Other bio-regulators have been described by Pogell (1979).

A-factor and related substances, the structures of which are now known, are attracting much interest. Gräfe *et al.* (1984) have studied the effect of bio-regulators that are related to A-factor and have observed their effect on the lipids of the cytoplasmic membrane. These are known to play an important role in differentiation. The evidence suggests that the pattern of differentiation is determined very early in the culture period. In this work also, submerged cultures were examined, and the bio-regulator was found to have a considerable effect. Khokhlov (1982) showed that A-factor has a considerable effect on streptomycin production in low-yielding mutants, but not on high yielders.

Genetic aspects of the production of A-factor in *S. coelicolor* have been investigated by Hara, Horinouchi & Uozumi (1983), and some of the genes involved have been mapped. It was noted that A-factor occurs in many species of *Streptomyces*. The general conclusion reached by these workers is that secondary metabolism forms part of the pattern of differentiation, either as a step in the process, or in association with a particular morphological step, such as occurs in the coloration of the spores of *S. coelicolor* at the completion of their formation.

Related work on the branching of *Achlya bisexualis* has been reported by Harold & Harold (1986). This shows that branching is enhanced by three classes of substances, cytochalasins A and E, a calcium ionophore, and two proton ionophores. It is considered that the effects of the cytochalasins reflect the disruption of the microfilament-based system of vesicle transport, and that the ionophores implicate cytoplasmic ions in branch initiation. These phenomena may be linked to an earlier discovery that a new point of proton entry precedes the emergence of a branch and predicts its locus. This paper provides a most useful review of modern work in this area of microbial physiology.

While these advances in the field of bio-regulation may seem to increase the complexity of the subject, they are of great significance in process development in stressing that there is a complex mechanism behind many of the cell processes, which, at present, often seem arbitrary and only to be understood empirically. An increasing knowledge of this area of research will lead to great advances in the theory of process development and the possibility of more systematic approaches.

Reverting to an older area of research, cases are known where the addition of specific chemicals can enhance the performance of antibiotic fermentations. Examples are the addition of tryptophane to cultures of *Claviceps* to increase the production of ergot (Robbers & Floss, 1976), or the addition of methionine to cultures of *Cephalosporium acremonium* to increase the formation of arthrospores and the production of cephalosporin C.

3.4.3   Differentiation in submerged culture

Owing to the type of growth that occurs in submerged culture, usually with the absence of sporulation, it is difficult to be clear about differentiation events, but it seems clear that it must be occurring in some form or another, especially in connection with the onset of secondary metabolism. Duckworth & Harris (1949) described a series of changes occurring in stirred penicillin production cultures, and other fermentations have been described. As growth and differentiation occur, a mixture of cell forms are present in the fermenter, resulting in changes in the pattern of pelleting, which thus affects viscosity and oxygen transfer. Changes in differentiation will therefore be important in fermentation optimisation. Differentiation seems to become less obvious in high-yielding mutants, compared with wild strains.

3.4.4   Relation to process development

Differentiation can thus be summarised as occurring in steps, with secondary metabolism commencing during one of these steps. This can be expressed:

differentiation steps

spores → 1   2   3   4   5   6 etc. → well-developed colony

secondary metabolism
commences

In submerged culture, a series of changes due to differentiation are usually observed, such as branching of the hyphae, formation of special types of pellets, secondary metabolism, fragmentation, and sometimes, in streptomycetes, the formation of spore-like bodies. It is not clear how these relate to the events seen in surface cultures.

It is clear that in industrial fermentations differentiation must be caused to occur in an optimal manner if maximum production is to be obtained. It is not possible to miss out steps in development, and, if the culture passes the desired stage of differentiation ineffectively, it is not possible to go back. Once the culture starts to go wrong, it may be impossible to reverse it.

The idea that the culture becomes active as regards antibiotic production and can remain so for a certain time is in agreement with these concepts. The object must be to move the culture into the productive phase and then, if possible, lock it into this condition, preventing further development steps. Additionally, the inoculation and initiation of the culture must be such that there is a good start to production. Unsuitable inoculum, at the wrong stage of differentiation, will produce poor results. It is known also that in some fermentations too rapid initial growth can disorganise the initial stages, so that secondary metabolism fails to start or is only transient. On the other hand, the correct form of pelleting in *Aspergillus niger* greatly increases citric acid production, an example of securing and holding a particular cell condition.

3.5   The oxytetracycline fermentation

The subject of oxytetracycline (OTC) production is introduced here, as a contrast to the penicillin fermentation which has already been discussed. This allows a comparison between the similarities and differences in the cases of the two fermentations, and the expansion of the area investigated. In this case, data is available from several fermentations, and these bring out the factors which become important as titres increase.

3.5.1   Fermentation methods

Oxytetracycline is produced by *Streptomyces rimosus* and some related species among the streptomycetes. The same fermenters were used as for penicillin, but it was necessary to reduce the rate of stirring to 520 rpm, and the airflow to 0.5 l/l/min. With the higher level of stirring and aeration, the culture grew very fast and showed only a poor degree of secondary metabolism. The production medium contained (g/l): starch, 63; soya bean meal, 7.5; corn-steep liquor, 12; $(NH_4)_2SO_4$, 5; $CaCO_3$, 23; NH_4Cl, 1.7; $KH_2PO_4 \cdot 4H_2O$, 0.05; polypropylene glycol 2500, 0.2; arachis oil, 20. The calcium carbonate used was Britomaya Violet Label (British Whiting Co., Melbourne, Herts.). The inoculum was prepared via the steps: spore suspension from a slope, shaken flask culture, stirred inoculum culture, with 300 ml of the latter being added to 2.7 l of production medium (Al-Jawadi, 1984; cf. Al-Jawadi & Calam, 1987).

Data from three oxytetracycline-producing strains or mutants are shown in Fig. 3.9a,b,c. Fig. 3.9d will be discussed later.

3.5.2   Patterns of growth and production

The curves for growth and production in Fig. 3.9a,b,c approximately follow the patterns observed with penicillin. There was a change from a restricted form of growth with the wild strain (72T1) to a smoother and

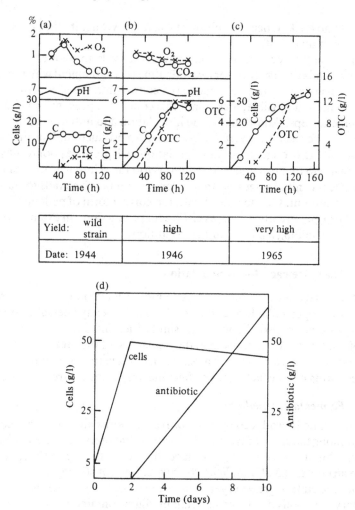

Fig. 3.9. Oxytetracycline: development of mutants and process. (a) 72T1; (b) Y20; (c) improved mutant; (d) modern maximal antibiotic batch (stylised). OTC, oxytetracycline.

more extended pattern in the mutants. The curves for the specific production rates are shown in Fig. 3.10, and these bring this out clearly. With the mutants, Q_{OTC} doubled, and the production period was extended to a marked extent. This explains the increase in production from 1 g/l to 12.5 g/l with the best strain.

With the wild strain, growth ceased sharply as early as 24 h, and there was a sharp break in growth and production with Y20 (Fig. 3.9b) at 90 h. This break, with Y20, was not due to a shortage of oxygen, as the DOT was over 50%, and the addition of starch or ammonium salts had no

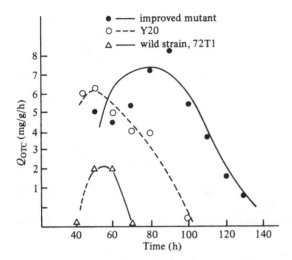

Fig. 3.10. Specific productivity of *S. rimosus* strains producing oxytetracycline (OTC).

effect. The cessation of growth and production must therefore have been due to the toxic effect of the oxytetracycline, this toxicity well known to be critical in this fermentation. With the improved mutant, growth and production continued longer, but production slowed down greatly after 120 h, indicating the effect of product toxicity.

3.5.3 Respiration and growth

There were considerable differences between the behaviour of the wild strain and the mutant Y20 (Fig. 3.9a,b). It is interesting to compare the respiratory behaviour of *S. rimosus* (Y20) with that of *P. chrysogenum*. As Y20 showed an RQ well below 1, and because RQ seemed to vary with *S. rimosus* strains, oxygen uptake was used directly as an indicator of the respiration rate. The results obtained are shown in Table 3.3, along with those from Run 30 for comparison.

The oxytetracycline fermentation used much less oxygen, largely because fewer cells were produced and because of the lower maintenance requirements. However, the requirement for cell growth was twice that for penicillin. This difference in requirements would have a considerable effect on the planning of a maximal oxytetracycline fermentation.

3.5.4 Morphological differences between strains in submerged culture

Differences in morphological behaviour between 72T1 and the mutant Y20 are shown in Fig. 3.11 (cf. Al-Jawadi & Calam, 1987). Information from samples was obtained using a scanning microscope. The figure also shows the growth, RQ, and specific production rate curves, for

Table 3.3. *Respiration data from penicillin and oxytetracycline batches*

Batch	Parameters			Cells produced (g/l)	Oxygen used (l)		
	Y	p	m		total	cells	maintenance
Penicillin (Run 30)	2.6	0.07	0.0065	50	58	17.5	41
Oxytetracycline (Y20)	1.3	0.05	0.002	28	24	17.2	6.5

comparision. With 72T1, the RQ fell steadily, showing marked changes in cell metabolism throughout.

The wild strain grew initially as fine hyphae, in loose pellets, which soon began to break down to spore-like bodies. Later some free particles were seen in the process of germination. There was thus an obvious pattern of differentiation. The effect of toxicity might have had an effect, as 72T1 was inhibited by oxytetracycline at 3 g/l (on agar), the mutant being much less sensitive, even at high concentrations. The Pfizer isolate, NRRL 2234, which produces oxytetracycline, showed comparable effects.

The mutant Y20 was much more stable morphologically, occurring as fine hyphae in loose pellets. Only at the end of the fermentation did some swellings appear in the hyphae, and a few globular bodies were seen.

3.6   Production of maximum yields

Information on the performance of modern oxytetracycline fermentations is not available, but Fig. 3.9d suggests the shape of the growth curve that is generally associated with maximum production of other antibiotics at the present time, with individual processes having their own characteristic forms. Just as Fig. 3.1 suggests material flows in cells in terms of a few arrows, Fig. 3.9d summarises the general production pattern in three straight lines. The main feature is growth reaching a maximum in 2 days, limited by the supply of phosphate, or other chosen element, with slowly declining cell concentration thereafter. Production starts during or at the end of the growth phase and continues for 7 or more days, with a constant value of Q_p, giving yields of 50–60 g/l or more. These curves were kindly made available by Dr I. S. Hunter, who used them to show the bi-phasic nature of antibiotic fermentations, as a background to a lecture on differential gene expression and the time-dependent synthesis of cloned genes.

It is evident that there are substantial differences, in principle, between the curves in Figs. 3.9d and 3.9c, and that the new form must involve a total replanning of the fermentation on a carefully worked-out basis. This, in relation to the main nutrient flows, will be discussed later. The

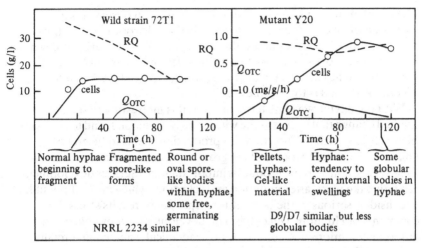

Fig. 3.11. Comparison of morphology between wild strain and mutant.

inorganic flow-system is also important. For example, microbial cells contain about 3% of phosphate (as P_2O_5). To meet this, the growth of 25 g/l of cells would need 1.4 g/l of KH_2PO_4, and 50 g/l of cells would need 2.8 g/l of KH_2PO_4, or more. These are values higher than those traditionally used in media. Cessation of growth due to a lack of inorganic constituents could be easily attributed to product inhibition. The treatment of this area of metabolism will have to be a matter of reflection on the part of the reader, as it forms a major subject in itself, if treated fully.

3.7   Discussion

The object of the present chapter has been to consider the antibiotic-producing culture as a physiological machine, and to indicate some of the main processes involved, as an aid to understanding fermentation work. These ideas will be extended further as the book proceeds.

The comparison of the penicillin and oxytetracycline fermentations shows similarities and differences and, especially with oxytetracycline, a tendency for minor factors to be important for success. This dependence of secondary metabolism on particular conditions is common among the bacteria. For example, the production of the red pigment prodigiosin by *Serratia marcescens* occurs in cultures at 25 °C but not at 37 °C, while pseudomonads produce yellow fluorescence in the presence of phosphate, though phosphate is not required for the production of the blue pigment pyocyanin, and cultures vary in their capacity to produce one or other of the pigments. The sorts of variation observed with oxytetracycline are similar, and workers in the field soon discover how to overcome them and to obtain stable behaviour. In considering the way a fermentation works, it is easy to overlook details of this kind; each fermentation has its own peculiarities, which have to be taken into account if success is to be achieved.

With the oxytetracycline fermentation, it is interesting to see the gradual change that occurs as the wild strain is developed, and to compare high-yielding fermentations, where production seems to be growth linked, with an ideal process where growth and production are separated. Clearly, resistance to the product is important here. Serious development can only take place after mutation and selection, which make it possible to consider, seriously, the best future steps. These results stress the comments of Huber & Teitz (1983) on development; they contrast the different conditions and cultures used academically and commercially, and the different types of information likely to come from them.

The initial theoretical conceptions applied to fermentations often seem static, while examples are mobile, constantly changing the perspectives they reveal, and suggesting areas where new ideas can be used. Anyone working in development research is likely to pick out his or her own points of maximum interest. Sometimes an answer can be found in a book, but it is usually best to create new answers, using the quickest and simplest methods.

When attempting to tackle a problem in process development, the first needs are to find out what is going on in the fermentation and what is limiting it, and then to form a view of what aspects are important and how they relate to each other, and to suggest a way ahead. What is written here shows that there is no one way, but the examples do give an opportunity to reconsider and to ask questions, such as: What are the key points? What information is missing? What are the next most useful steps? Finding the questions and the answers is the first step for the expert. The examples are also useful in showing the sort of data usually available and ways to make the best use of it. Looking at this another way, if the data are found to be inconsistent or not fit the expected pattern, it may mean that there has been an error, or that the outlook of the expert is mistaken or too limited. Experts are as much individuals as are fermentations. It is not surprising that their questions and answers also differ.

These and other matters will be considered in more detail as the book continues. Many subjects have not yet been touched upon, and the illogical and complicated aspects of the subject have not yet been introduced. The subject of microbial physiology is so large that only a fraction can be seen. It is only possible to provide a few pegs on which ideas can be hung, with a few to spare to accommodate novel ideas arising from new research.

4 Microbial biochemistry

Biochemistry attempts a detailed analysis of the reaction sequences important in growth and biosynthesis and the ways in which they are regulated. It is also concerned with the chemical substances involved. These biochemical reactions are all brought about by biological catalysts, i.e. the enzymes. The synthesis of these enzymes and its regulation are brought about by the nucleus and are therefore under genetic control. Thus the combined biochemical–genetic system is central whenever consideration is given to microbial behaviour. The subject is therefore extensive and complex. Those interested should consult a suitable textbook, such as Conn & Stumpf's *Outlines of Biochemistry* (1976). However, caution is needed because there are differences between animal and microbial biochemistry, as well as differences between eukaryotic and prokaryotic biochemistry.

4.1 Enzyme reactions

The basis of life processes is the existence of enzymes – catalysts that accelerate chemical reactions leading to the production of substances, with large or small molecules, that are the basis of cell structures and cell metabolism.

Important features of living cells are (1) the large number of enzymes commonly involved, perhaps 2000 or more, (2) the existence of chain reactions in which enzymes work together, and (3) the close control of these systems which is exerted at different levels. In development work, increases in production seem to be brought about mainly by alterations to these regulatory systems.

Consider, for instance, the formation of acetoacetate from acetate. This can be carried out chemically by heating ethyl acetate with sodium, which catalyses a multi-step reaction. Enzymically it is produced by a complex reaction that carboxylates the acetyl units to malonyl units, pairs of which are then condensed and decarboxylated. Chemical and biochemical reactions seem alike, but this is incorrect, since biochemically the acetyl units must be activated by combination with coenzyme-A (a reaction requiring ATP) and, in any case, the whole system is controlled genetically, the enzyme concentration and its activity being adjusted to meet the requirements of the cell.

The biosynthesis of intermediate substances and cell products are brought about by chains of reactions, each step requiring the action of an enzyme. Such a chain might be written:

$$
\begin{array}{c}
\text{G} \\
\searrow \\
\text{A} \rightarrow \text{B} \rightarrow \text{C} \rightarrow \text{D} \rightarrow \text{E} \rightarrow \text{F} \\
\searrow \\
\text{H}
\end{array}
$$

in which the substance A is converted to F by a series of five enzymes. As indicated, such a chain may be involved with other chains, with one or more of the intermediates supplying these other routes. In the diagram, the enzymes are indicated as arrows, pointing in one direction. In fact, enzyme reactions may go one way or both ways, or both-way reactions may occur because of the presence of two separate enzymes that probably have different characteristics. As with the case of malonyl production, described above, some of the enzyme steps may seem simple, but they are actually complex reactions in themselves.

In many cases, starting materials and intermediates require activation before reactions can occur. This activation usually involves a coenzyme, for example coenzyme-A (a thiol derivative of pantothenic acid and adenosine diphosphate), while other substances are activated by phosphation. Other substances are involved as carriers, for example ATP (adenosine triphosphate), which carries energy, and NAD (nicotinamide adenine dinucleotide), which transfers H^+ in oxidation–reduction reactions.

In the cell, the enzymes may occur as colloidal particles in the cytoplasm, but most are attached to membranes in the cell. In some cases, such as the synthesis of fatty acids and some antibiotics, the group of enzymes required is located on a large protein template of high molecular weight ($1-1.5 \times 10^6$).

4.2   Regulation of enzyme reactions

The rate of enzyme reactions are regulated in three main ways: by the concentration of the substrate; by feedback mechanisms; and, genetically, by mRNA transcription.

Concentration of substrate
The relation between the reaction rate and the substrate concentration (S) is expressed by the equation:

$$
\text{rate} = \text{rate}_{max}\left(\frac{S}{S + K_m}\right)
$$

where K_m, the Michaelis constant, is the value of S when the rate falls to half the maximum. With an expression of this sort, the rate is independent of S until S falls to a low level, when the rate declines rapidly.

The Michaelis constant is also referred to as the affinity coefficient. When K_m is high, the affinity of the substrate to the enzyme is low, and vice versa. This is a useful concept, especially when considering the behaviour of two enzymes, with different affinities, competing for a particular substrate.

Feedback mechanisms
In a typical enzyme chain, such as that depicted above, the reaction rate is controlled by feedback provided by the concentration of the product (F). This is brought about because as the concentration rises, the shape of the first enzyme in the chain (A $\rightarrow$ B) changes so as to reduce its action, this being referred to as allosteric control. This effect goes much further than feedback in an individual chain, since often an allosteric enzyme is affected by related substances and by different substances. Thus, the tricarboxylic acid (TCA) cycle is extensively regulated by the concentration of ATP on certain of the enzymes, thus regulating the production of energy in relation to the demand on the system.

Regulation by mRNA transcription
Enzymes are essentially unstable, having half-lives of hours in prokaryotes (less than an hour in some cases) and 1–2 days in eukaryotes. Thus, as the enzymes decay, the level of their product falls and the reaction slows down. The concentration of the enzyme may therefore need to be restored. The enzymes are synthesised on the ribosomes, on the basis of copies of the relevant section of the nucleus, which are transferred thither by messenger RNA (mRNA). These copies are made by short strands of mRNA, which scan the nucleus and transcribe sections that are open for copying. The genes involved with a group of enzymes producing a particular substance are arranged in groups referred to as operons. These operons include three regulatory genes, as well as the genes controlling enzyme synthesis. These regulatory genes are the promoter, giving the location for copying, a regulator, and an operator, which is sensitive to the product and which makes the operon sensitive or insensitive for copying.

This brief account gives a working outline of the principles of cell regulation. To grasp its complexity and flexibility, a detailed study would be necessary if an idea of what is involved is to be obtained. It may be mentioned that the promoter and its location has a great effect on the productivity of the operon, and this aspect is important in strain development by mutation, especially in direct gene transfer techniques. It should be stressed that regulation, in the sense of the induction and repression of enzyme reactions, can be brought about in many ways; for example, penicillin production can be repressed by the presence of penicillin itself, or by the presence of lysine, an amino acid that tends to accumulate in the medium (Demain, 1957). Many biosyntheses are repressed by glucose or phosphate. For an account of regulation in microbial systems and antibiotic production, see Martin & Demain (1980) and Demain (1982).

4.3   Central metabolism and its regulation

The glycolysis–tricarboxylic acid cycle system provides a central pathway in cell metabolism, from which branch more-specific biosynthetic functions, and by which energy is supplied. It has been extensively studied and is under constant reconsideration. The system operates in different forms in prokaryotes, the fungi, plants, and animals. The last three, being eukaryotic, have the energy-producing system in the mitochondrion, which has its own subsidiary genetic control unit, and this involves mechanisms for the transfer of material into and out of this organelle. This tends to produce a more-complicated arrangement than that in prokaryotes.

Fig. 4.1 gives an outline of the pathways of central metabolism as found in bacteria, based on the work of Weitzman (1981). It shows the main nutrients (in boxes) entering from the top and from the left- and right-hand sides.

The chart shows three or four main areas. On the left, carbohydrates enter as C_6PO_4 compounds, via the glycolytic pathway. As media for antibiotic production usually contain protein and vegetable oil these are shown entering from the top; the amino acids enter via ketoglutarate, and the fatty acids enter by acetyl-CoA in the central area. In this system the central area of supplementary metabolism is stressed. Glucogenesis can occur via oxalacetate (OAA) and phosphoenolpyruvate (PEP). When modelling the griseofulvin fermentation (Calam *et al.*, 1971), it was found that considerable glucogenesis was necessary to provide for the observed cell growth, and this is probably necessary in many other cases.

It will be seen here that the TCA cycle is acting in three different ways: energy generation, catabolism enabling the input of material for metabolism, and provision of starting points for biosynthesis. Examples of this are shown in the synthesis of amino acids and of malonyl units, the starting points for many antibiotics.

Energy formation commences with the synthesis of acetyl-CoA, at the beginning of the TCA cycle, which then combines with oxalacetate (OAA) to form citrate. The TCA cycle is shown in Fig. 4.1 as a circle. Two acetyl-CoA units are formed per molecule of glucose, each unit being subsequently decomposed in the cycle to carbon dioxide, giving rise to

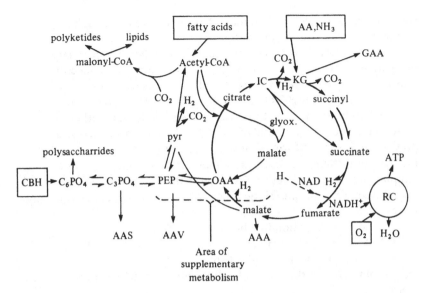

Fig. 4.1. Outline of central metabolism. The main inputs, carbohydrates (CBH), fatty acids, ammonia (NH_3), amino acids (AA), and O_2, are shown in boxes. The location of synthesis of amino acids is shown: AAA, aspartic, asparagine, threonine, methionine and nucleotides; GAA, glutamic, glutamine, proline, arginine, lysine, amino-adipic acid; AAS, serine, cysteine, tryptophane; AAV, valine, alanine, leucine. C_3PO_4, C_6PO_4, tri- and hexa-phospho carbohydrates; glyox., glyoxalate; pyr, pyruvate; RC, respiratory centre; KG, ketoglutarate; IC, isocitrate; OAA, oxalacetate; PEP, phosphoenol pyruvate.

electrons. These are, in turn, taken up by NAD to form $NADH^+$. The $NADH^+$ units pass to the respiratory system, yielding NAD, water, and energy conserved as ATP. Two ATP units are produced by glycolysis, and a further 36 are produced by the TCA cycle, i.e. 18 per acetyl unit. This is if respiration is efficient. With bakers' yeast, the P/O ratio is 2 instead of 3, and even lower yields may occur. As mentioned previously, the rate of energy formation is governed by the level of ATP in the system. Low levels stimulate pyruvate dehydrogenase, citrate synthase, oxyglutarate dehydrogenase, and isocitrate dehydrogenase, and also glycolysis, thus increasing cycle activity, while high levels depress the system. In this way, multi-point control is secured. It is also referred to as energy charge control.

4.4 Biosynthesis of microbial products

As mentioned above, the starting points for biosynthesis of antibiotics may be sugars, amino acids, malonyl-CoA units, and acetoacetate units. The isoprenoids are formed from acetyl-CoA or leucine, via a complex route through mevalonic acid to 2,3-dimethylallyl pyrophosphate, the unit forming the basis for biosynthesis.

Since so many antibiotics are produced, a corresponding variety of biosyntheses are involved. The antibiotics are, however, concentrated into a relatively few categories, such as the amino-sugar-based antibiotics like streptomycin, the β-lactam antibiotics formed from amino acids, and the polyketides such as the tetracyclines, macrolides, and others.

In each category, the initial building blocks are synthesised and polymerised, so as to form an initial precursor (such as methyl-pre-tetramid in the tetracyclines). In this stage an enzyme template may be employed. Subsequently the precursor is modified and substituted to give the antibiotic. The process thus involves the following stages.

(1) Formation of building blocks.
(2) Assembly to give precursor.
(3) Final modification and substitution.

Details of the biosynthesis of individual antibiotics will be found in the literature.

It will be appreciated that each stage of the process involves a complex series of events, and that the biosynthetic process forms part of the metabolic system of the cells, which depends on materials obtained from central metabolism. Faults in the planning of the fermentation can lead to a lack of particular intermediates, resulting in reduced biosynthesis. The assembly of the building blocks and their polymerisation takes place in a particular order, commencing with the starter unit. This often differs from the others, for example in the tetracyclines the starter is a molecule of amido-malonyl-CoA. The formation of this requires special biosynthetic steps. If amido-malonyl-CoA is not available, the organism uses acetoacetyl-CoA, which gives a different product of low activity, acetyltetracycline. In some of the macrolides, the starters are quite complex substances, and the polymerisation involves propionyl as well as acetyl units.

The final stage will require a number of modifications to the structure and the introduction of new groupings. There is obviously the possibility of variations, giving rise to different products. Examples are tetracycline, chlortetracycline, oxytetracycline, and demethyl-tetracycline, each showing a minor change. A product may require more than one type of building block; mycophenolic acid involves a polyketide unit plus an isoprenoid side chain. Biosynthesis also requires energy; 1 g of penicillin requires 2.1–2.2 l of oxygen for this purpose.

4.5   Mechanistic model of antibiotic production

Having described physiological aspects of the cell mechanism, it is interesting to consider a general model of antibiotic production, on the

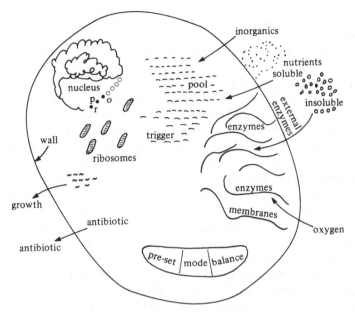

Fig. 4.2. General model of cell mechanism. Conditions to be optimised: pH, concentrations, dissolve oxygen, mixing, morphology, K_{La}.

basis of the information presented in Figs. 3.1 and 4.1, which summarise some of the main mechanisms involved, Fig. 3.1 describes material flows, and Fig. 4.1 describes the biochemistry involved, from which key reactions could be chosen. Experimental data could be used to define these matters in more detail, if a quantitative model was being prepared. The model would have to take into account: (1) utilisation of nutrients and oxygen, (2) production and maintenance of cells, (3) the production of antibiotic and other substances.

Fig. 4.2 gives a general idea of the cell as a reactive system. It incorporates some of the main features so far described, such as the nucleus, with an operon with regulator, operator, and promoter genes (r, o, p), along with some ribosomes to represent the regulatory chain. Organic and inorganic nutrients and oxygen enter the cell, forming a pool containing the materials needed for metabolism. The enzymes are also indicated, and it is assumed that the majority would be attached to membranes within the cell. The production of antibiotic is shown, and the accumulation of material for growth is indicated. It is assumed that carbon dioxide is also being liberated.

Fig. 4.2 also tries to bring out that the cells can exist in different states, by the words pre-set, mode, and balance. Thus the cells are pre-set by the inoculum, are triggered into modes by differentiation, and are affected by the balance of conditions in the fermenter and the cells themselves. It is assumed that these conditions will be optimised for maximum production, but this is not always achieved.

It is not proposed here to develop this material into a quantitative model, as to do so would require a great deal of space and involve a mass of detail. Anyone who wishes to do so would find it a matter of the greatest interest and would gain a considerable insight into fermentation work. Details of a number of fermentations that could provide a basis are given in this book. A simpler type of model is described in Chapter 8.

A model of the griseofulvin fermentation was developed by Calam, Ellis & McCann (1971), much on the lines described here, using a systems engineering approach. It was found necessary to greatly limit the amount of detail incorporated into the model. This included 17 reactions, which covered the fermentation fairly well. It was impossible to control the model by Michaelis-type regulation, and many restrictions had to be included to secure an orderly metabolic pattern. These restrictions appeared to represent the regulatory action of the nucleus.

A study of the model led to the impression that the fermentation consists of a complex reaction system subject to an elaborate, double control system. This mechanism is sensitive to current conditions, but its behaviour is affected considerably by what has gone before, during the fermentation. To an extent, the problem in fermentation development work is as much to do with optimising these internal control mechanisms as it is to do with optimising the biosynthetic chains.

On thinking over the subject, it becomes apparent, in the first place, that the system is a very complicated one, and even with a powerful modelling language and a large computer, it is difficult to fully realise the concepts involved. At the same time, on looking at the sort of biochemical skeleton that can be constructed (e.g. Fig. 3.1), it is apparent that it involves only a few percent of the reactions occurring in the cells, and that we are still ignorant of many of the principles involved, or, at least, of how to express them adequately. Thus, the sort of biochemical model that can be developed is too elementary to be very helpful. Although this may seem contradictory and pessimistic, it brings out the exciting challenges that exist in this area of microbiology.

5 Subsidiary factors important in production fermentations

Several antibiotic fermentations have been discussed and illustrated by curves of growth and production, and the impression has probably been given that it is easy to obtain good results. In fact, it is not difficult to obtain good results, but many beginners find it hard at first. This is because it is always essential, if good results are to be obtained, to use optimal growth conditions and to inoculate with a culture in perfect condition for the job. Achieving this condition may be easy or difficult, depending on the strain being used, but it always requires attention. For optimal production it is usually also necessary to meet a number of special conditions during the fermentation; the importance of these conditions may be unexpected.

These subsidiary factors therefore deserve attention. The subject is difficult because the critical factors differ for each fermentation and have to be worked out by experience. This chapter will therefore give a number of illustrative examples that demonstrate the kind of details likely to need consideration.

The fact that it is necessary to have all stages of the inoculum in the right condition suggests that cell differentiation is the key factor (see Chapter 3.6). However, too little is known at present to be certain of the exact way differentiation brings about the observed effects, and an empirical approach is necessary.

Development work usually means testing various fermentation procedures so as to obtain the best results. These tests can only be useful if all conditions are optimal. The basic process itself must be optimised, and all subsidiary factors, such as the inoculum, must be adjusted to give ideal conditions. Tests under conditions giving low yields, or far from the industrial process, are unlikely to be of much significance.

5.1   Effect of preparation of the inoculum

Experience with different filamentous organisms may be mentioned briefly.

Results with *Penicillium chrysogenum* JV 101 in shaken culture with corn-steep medium (Smith & Calam, 1980) are summarised in Table 5.1. The growth pattern is also affected by the type of medium, as shown by experiments with *Aspergillus oryzae* (Table 5.2). The effect went

57

Table 5.1. *Spore concentration in inoculum and penicillin production*

Spores in inoculum/ml	10^2	10^3	2×10^3	10^4
Growth in production flasks	dense pellets	dense pellets	open pellets	filaments
Penicillin (max. u/ml)	500	1800	4000	5000

Table 5.2. *Growth pattern and medium*

Spore conc./ml	2×10^4	2×10^5	10^6
Synthetic medium	pellets	pellets	filaments
Synthetic medium + CSL and CaCO$_3$	filaments and pellets	filaments	filaments

Table 5.3. *Penicillin: pellet sizes in shaken-flask production cultures*

Age (h)	Percentage of pellets with size ranges (mm diameter)						Average size of pellet (mm diameter)
	0–0.9	1–1.9	2–2.9	3–3.9	4–4.9	5–5.9	
1. Spores (inoculum), 10^3/ml; penicillin, 2100 u/ml							
0	87	13					0.7
27	50	48	2				1.2
47	9	58	31	2			1.9
54	6	40	51	3			2.0
78		4	41	54	3		3.0
124			2	31	56	11	4.2
2. Spores (inoculum), 10^4/ml; penicillin, 5050 u/ml							
0	99	1					0.4
27	7	89	5				1.3
47	27	63	9				1.2
54	32	62	5				1.2
78	51	36	14				1.1
124	72	27	1				0.8

somewhat deeper than might be judged by appearance, since dense pellets could be obtained that failed to grow further when inoculated into a second-stage culture.

In shaken flasks there is a considerable wall effect, as clumps of spores appear to move into a ring just above the level of the swirling liquid; these then fall back into the medium and form pellets or filaments, depending on the number of spores in the clumps. It was found that with *Penicillium stoloniferum*, ring formation could be prevented by adding small glass floats, to bring the spores back into the medium to give filamentous growth. If ring formation was allowed to start, repeated removal of the ring with a sterile swab could remove all the spores from the flask.

These results show that the process of spore clumping and of later development is a complicated process. This means that if inocula are grown in stirred culture, the results with a given medium may differ from those produced in shaken culture.

As mentioned in Chapter 2, the pellets formed under different conditions can be classified as dense, open, or filamentous, each category including quite different culture forms. Thus pellet types can be associated with different degrees of productivity. One of the best-studied areas here is in connection with the production of citric acid. There have been a number of publications in this field; small pellets, 0.5 mm diameter, consisting of radiating and thickened hyphae are mentioned as optimal by Miles Laboratories Inc. (1952). The impression is that with different citric-acid-producing strains the optimal types of pellets differ, and that the best conditions for citric acid production also vary between strains.

Thus, pellet formation involves not only the idea of the production of an optimal kind of mycelium, but also a particular physiological and biochemical state, which has to be exploited in a particular way to give optimal results. While with some species of microorganisms this can be critical, in others it may be much less so. This can only be determined by experience.

Pellets grow in different ways. This is illustrated by data obtained using *P. chrysogenum* JV 101, shown in Table 5.3. It is seen that with a production culture started with an inoculum seeded with 10^3 spores/ml the pellets grew larger, while with 10^4 spores/ml in the inoculum the tiny pellets remained small but became more numerous.

The manner in which productivity was fixed by the state of the inoculum was shown by an experiment in which pellets were homogenised (Smith & Calam, 1980). The results are given in Table 5.4. The experiment shows that although homogenisation broke up the pellets and produced filamentous growth in the production stage, penicillin production remained sub-optimal, at about half the maximum level. It is evident that

Table 5.4. *Effect of homogenisation on production*

Time blended (sec)	Penicillin (u/ml)	Appearance at end of production phase
0	400	large pellets
20	1400	medium pellets
90	2450	filaments
180	2800	filaments

Control: 5000 u/ml.

the hyphae had been produced in an inefficient state, and that this continued during the production stage.

The linkage between the form of the pellets and their biochemical properties is shown by the experiments described in Table 5.5, based on data from Smith & Calam (1980). The mycelium from the production cultures was assayed for certain key enzymes (ICDH, G6PDH). The relationships between enzyme activities and productivity are well shown. The difference in enzyme activities show the biochemical difference between the cultures, though its connection with productivity is not known.

5.2   Fixation of inoculum quality

The point at which the desired form of inoculum culture became fixed, to give maximum yields, was determined by inoculating a suitably high concentration of spores of *P. chrysogenum* JV 101 into inoculum medium, incubating on the shaker, and then diluting the suspension at intervals to a sub-optimal concentration, 10^3/ml. The inocula produced with the diluted spores were then added to production medium after 40 h of growth (Calam & Smith, 1981). The results are summarised in Table 5.6. With dilution up to 20 h, productivity was low and large pellets were formed. The period 20–30 h marked a transitional stage, before a later stage when the inoculum behaved as a high-spore-concentration culture. During the intermediate period, the flasks showed no growth, and the mycelium consisted of very short threads, with only a few branches, at most. It is evident that the factors that produce particular types of pelleting are operating before the pellets appear. Hence, they are not mainly physiological factors such as lack of oxygen or nutrients, as these will not yet have developed in the culture.

This study of inoculum cultures stresses an important aspect of antibiotic fermentations. As a rule, the fermentations show a number of growth phases, for example initial rapid growth leading to periods of

Table 5.5. *Enzyme activities and data from production cultures*

Inoculum spore conc. (spores/ml)	Inoculum (40 h)	Production culture at			
		24 h	48 h	96 h	120 h
		Dry weight (g/l)			
1×10^3	2.7	6	9	15.5	17
5×10^3	3.7	7	11	23	28
1×10^4	10	11.5	15.5	27	28
5×10^4	12.9	14	17.5	28	28
		Penicillin (u/ml)			
1×10^3	—	30	50	780	900
5×10^3	—	60	140	3000	4800
1×10^4	—	120	400	3500	5000
5×10^4	—	150	470	4000	5000
		ICDH activity (mU/mg dry cells)			
1×10^3	10	8	15	9	12
5×10^3	14	11	12	25	35
1×10^4	22	18	19	16	27
5×10^4	25	20	20	14	9
		G6PDH activity (mU/mg dry cells)			
1×10^3	12	12	13	12	11
5×10^3	42	21	25	16	15
1×10^4	62	36	28	10	5
5×10^4	69	38	26	7	5

Table 5.6. *Effects of dilution on inoculum quality*

Age when diluted (h)	Penicillin (u/ml at 5 days)	Morphological appearance of cultures	
		inoculum	production
0	1825	LCP	LCP
12	2125	LCP	LCP
20	2225	LCP	LCP
24	2850	SOP	SF
28	3325	SOP	SF
36	4375	SF	SFF
40	4700	SF	SFF
Control 10^5	4875	SF	SFF
Control 10^3	1820	LCP	LCP

LCP, large compact pellets; SOP, small open pellets; SF, small pellets and some filaments; SFF, filaments and a few small pellets.

Table 5.7. *Oxytetracycline fermentation: effect of chalk and inoculum*

Inoculum		Production		Product	
method	chalk	method	chalk	OTC	acetyl-OTC
shaken	A	shaken	A	+ +	+
stirred	B	stirred	B	+ + +	−
stirred	B	shaken	A	+ + +	−
shaken	A	stirred	B	+ + +	−
shaken	C	shaken	C	+ + +	−

slower growth, limited by nutrient or oxygen supply, or by product toxicity. During these stages the culture is adapting to the new conditions and producing the antibiotic. Ideally, the culture should act as an immobilised enzyme system, biosynthesising steadily throughout the fermentation, regardless of the changes taking place. Thus the pellets produced by the inoculum culture hold the keys to excellence in production. This emphasises the view that once a production culture is inoculated, it can be made worse but not better.

5.3   Inoculum quality and medium components in oxytetracycline production

When working on the oxytetracycline (OTC) fermentation, in shaken and stirred culture, several types of chalk ($CaCO_3$) were tested for their suitability; three samples, A, B and C, were used (Al-Jawadi, 1984). It is known that the quality of chalk is important in this fermentation, though the reason is unknown. It was found that shaken cultures usually gave oxytetracycline together with 33% of acetyl-oxytetracycline as an impurity, while stirred cultures gave only oxytetracycline. The results of the trials with the different chalks and fermentation conditions are summarised in Table 5.7.

Although there are gaps in the information, there is clearly an interaction between the type of chalk and the condition of culture. The use of stirred culture avoided the production of acetyl-OTC, i.e. oxytetracycline with an acetyl instead of the acetamide side chain usually present, while the use of chalk C prevented this, even in shaken culture. This is an example of the unexpected effects that can occur in antibiotic fermentations.

5.4   Initial growth rate in production cultures

There is a considerable amount of evidence that in production cultures the initial growth rate can have an important effect on the yield of antibiotic, although this is restricted to rather few published examples.

With penicillin production, L. D. Shtoffer (1978, personal communication) showed that with specific growth rates (μ) above 0.06 there was a tendency for yields to be reduced. Nelligan & Calam (1983) have confirmed this in fed-batch cultures grown on semi-synthetic medium. With $\mu = 0.10$, metabolism proved less efficient, with a lower yield of cells per litre of oxygen used. Production, though rapid at first, tended to fade rather quickly. This effect is not harmful in commercial batches aimed at a short fermentation time, when vigorous initial growth leads to a high production rate per litre, giving a high output in 4–5 days. Nelligan found that with a lower initial value for μ, production continued longer. It is interesting that even with the higher growth rate, penicillin still appeared at the normally expected time.

In the case of oxytetracycline production in stirred culture, as already described (Chapter 3.5), it was necessary to reduce the rate of stirring and aeration below that used for penicillin production to obtain satisfactory synthesis of oxytetracycline. The reason for this is unknown, but it appeared that if growth and respiration were too rapid, then induction of secondary metabolism was inhibited.

Vaněk & Hošťálek (1973) have also shown that in the production of chlortetracycline by *S. aureofaciens* it is advantageous to control the initial growth rate. This they did by addition of benzyl thiocyanate, a substance which restricts glycolysis, to mutant 84/25, which gave 4.5 g/l of chlortetracycline.

5.5   **Discussion**

The various effects described may seem rather irrational, but they do, in fact, seriously affect antibiotic fermentations, in some way or another. They emphasise that the fermentation starts with the spores used for inoculation and continues through the various stages until the completion of the production stage, as a continuous whole. Each step must be optimised, not only the medium and conditions, but all aspects of culture management. This is, in fact, usually achieved industrially, and once the key facts are known, a fair degree of consistency can be obtained. It is a matter that has to be taken into account when setting up a fermentation in the development laboratory, and it may require a considerable effort, so as to achieve a consistent performance and to deal with the varying quality of raw materials that are used in the medium.

Considering all the problems mentioned, to the newcomer it might seem that it would be difficult to achieve a successful fermentation without a good deal of trouble. As a rule, several things can simplify the problem. Firstly, when a new isolate is being used, the isolation system should include at least one medium, preferably of the complex type, that can form a basis for development. Secondly, experience is usually enough to ensure that reliable culture systems are used, with plenty of spores for seeding providing good growth in the inoculum stages, and reliable fermenter units are usually available. On these bases, it is usually possible to set up an adequate basic fermentation.

In this chapter, the emphasis has mainly been on the effect of the starting conditions on productivity. The interaction between the various forces that can act on the culture and that arise from the initial conditions and from changes occurring as the cells grow will be considered in the next chapter.

6 Submerged culture conditions: the interaction between environment and genotype

6.1 Introduction

In an antibiotic fermentation, a culture is grown in a fermenter, in a medium that is usually supplemented by a nutrient feed. Success depends on the intrinsic activity of the cells and the obtaining of an adequate match between organism and conditions. The fermentation process is not a simple one, however; during production the conditions are continuously changing, and the cells are responding to these changes. The nucleus, it is true, remains the same, but it obviously operates in different modes, as evinced by the way in which the cells differentiate and develop during the growth cycle.

This interaction between organism and conditions has been expressed by the statement:

$$\text{phenotype} = \text{genotype} + \text{environment} \qquad (6.1)$$

This statement tends to be seen as static, but in fermentations it must be seen as mobile, with all three components changing due to the interactions caused by the processes of metabolism.

The changes that occur in cell metabolism, as growth proceeds, are illustrated, for example, by the changing concentrations of enzymes in the mycelium in chlortetracycline fermentations (Hošťálek & Vaněk, 1973), by the micro-cycle (Smith & Galbraith, 1971), and by the work of Carter & Bull (1969) on the production of melanin by *Aspergillus nidulans*. Trigger effects and transcription regulation are both likely to be involved in these effects. To illustrate this further, some examples of antibiotic fermentations will be given in more detail. Although this subject is ill defined, it is important conceptually in development work, as it stresses the forces involved in the achievement of high yields.

6.2 Environment and genotype
6.2.1 Environment
In the fermenter, some of the main factors are the following.
  (a) The medium, containing the basic ingredients, plus any feeds used during the fermentation.
  (b) The temperature.
  (c) The degree and type of aeration and mixing, which determine the activity of the culture and the rate of oxygen supply.

65

(d) The cell concentration and the type of growth, which determine the thickness and viscosity of the culture and thereby reduce the effectiveness of the stirrer system.
(e) The accumulation of toxic or inhibitory substances, which can also restrict the fermentation.

6.2.2   Genotype

The genotype represents the particular genetic structure of the strain being used in the process. For each antibiotic, there will be a particular genotype, from which a family of mutants will descend. For mutants being developed in industrial laboratories, the genotypes will be different. Each manufacturer will have its own family of genotypes.

This matters in practice. The various families will differ in their reactions to the environments they are exposed to, resulting in different types of pelleting and biochemistry. As a result, optimisation will require, in each case, different fermentation conditions. This must be recognised, as confusion can occur if each set of mutants is expected to be the same.

6.3   Environment, genotype, and production

6.3.1   Effect of culture conditions

From the foregoing, it would be expected that if an antibiotic-producing mutant was grown under different conditions, different results (i.e. phenotypes) would be obtained. In the case of oxytetracycline, this has been illustrated by a comparison of stirred and shaken cultures (Chapter 5.3). In the case of penicillin, Fig. 6.1 shows the results obtained with two mutants in standard stirred fermenters, stirred at different rates, so as to give increasing rates of respiration (Calam, Driver & Bowers, 1951). These results emphasise that if efficient fermenters are to be used, mutants that will take advantage of the new conditions must be chosen.

6.3.2   Temperature: example of investigation of effect on penicillin production

Antibiotic fermentations are usually run at temperatures in the range 24–28 °C. There is often a fairly distinct optimal value, which in the case of penicillin, is 25–27 °C, with a sharp fall above 30 °C. While this value is important physiologically, it is also important in connection with the cooling of the fermenter. This cooling may be difficult with these relatively low temperatures. Early experience with the penicillin fermentation tended to suggest that the optimal temperatures for growth and penicillin production might be different. Owen & Johnson (1955), using shaken-flask trials, found that increased yields could be obtained by starting at 30 °C during the main growth phase, and using 20 °C during the

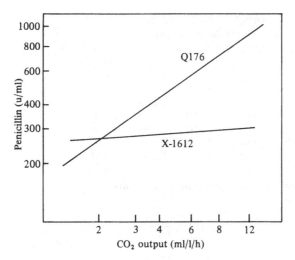

Fig. 6.1. Penicillin production by two mutants.

production phase. There is little doubt that, industrially, the optimisation of temperature profiles during antibiotic fermentations is taken very seriously.

Constantinides, Spencer & Gaden (1970) used experimental results from laboratory fermenters and plant trials to re-investigate the optimal temperature profile for penicillin production. The results confirmed those of Owen & Johnson (1955), but the work was mainly intended as an investigation of the application of mathematical optimisation techniques to a fermentation process, temperature being a convenient basis for study. The papers are mainly statistical, and difficult for microbiologists to understand, but they make an excellent starting point in this area of work. For the microbiologist, the manner of expressing fermentation patterns by a simple model is itself useful as a technique; it is also useful here, to show how patterns change in response to environment. Part of the data used has also been published (McCann & Calam, 1972), so that this adds an extra dimension to the example.

To apply the optimisation system to the batch results, it was necessary to express the growth and penicillin curves in a very few parameters. These were obtained by curve fitting, using the model equations given in Table 6.1. These make use of the logistic law equation for growth, and another equation, with two components (one relates production to cell concentration, and the other allows for the chemical destruction of penicillin in the medium). These parameters are defined in Table 6.1 by the terms k_1, x_{max}, k_2, and k_3. The values for the different temperatures are shown in Table 6.1, along with the penicillin production figures at 140 h.

Table 6.1. *Modelling the effect of temperature on penicillin production: changes in parameters*

Temp. (°C)	k_1	x_{max}	k_2	k_3	Penicillin, 140 h (u/ml)
18.2	0.31	47.7	3.37	0.013	5010
22.0	0.41	43.3	9.27	0.040	9390
25.0	0.55	40.2	14.00	0.056	10090
27.2	0.62	39.0	16.06	0.063	10380
30.3	0.38	41.8	10.25	0.055	6630

X = cell conc. (g/l); p = penicillin conc. (u/ml).
Equations used:

$$dx/dt = k_1 \cdot x\left(1 - \frac{x}{x_{max}}\right)$$
$$dp/dt = k_2 \cdot x - k_3 \cdot p$$

From the point of view of the present discussion, the important feature is the difference between the sets of parameters for each temperature, showing that, basically, the metabolism was different in each case. These differences are also apparent in the data presented by McCann & Calam (1972). These results also show the value of using simple models to express fermentation patterns in a simple and effective way. It is evident that equations of these kinds can be handled by computer, iteratively, over 10- or 5-h periods, with little difficulty.

6.3.3   The effect of loss of aeration and agitation

Fermentations sometimes break down after a good start. A common cause of this is a temporary failure of the agitation–aeration system, causing a temporary lack of oxygen. Another cause is that an infection may have occurred.

The subject was investigated by Hošťálek (1964) in shaken cultures of *S. aureofaciens* that produced chlortetracycline. The shaker was stopped for 10 min, each hour, over 6-h periods. The production levels achieved are summarised in Table 6.2, which also gives normal growth and production data for these conditions.

The greatest effect of the stoppages was at 6–12 h, which was part of the period of maximum cell activity, i.e. 12–24 h (Hošťálek & Vaněk, 1973). Tests made by Hošťálek (1964) showed that the effect of the cut in agitation was the loss of pentose-pathway activity, essential for maximum biosynthesis. Examination of the growth data shows that at the time in question (6–12 h) only a very small quantity of cells had been formed, but the damage persisted for a long time during growth. This example is of particular interest because the biochemistry of the effect was identified.

Table 6.2. *Effect of stoppages on chlortetracycline production in shaken flasks, and growth and production patterns*

Period of stoppages (10 min/h)	0–6	6–12	12–18	18–24	
Relative yield (% of normal)	95	35	43	75	
Normal data					
Age (h)	6	12	24	48	72
Cells (g/l)	2	3	8	13.5	14
Chlortetra-cycline (g/l)	0	0.1	0.25	1.0	1.6

Similar effects are observed with most other antibiotic fermentations. In other cases, such as yeast growth, stoppages also cause damage. In screening penicillin mutants, a stoppage of more than 5 min will render a batch of flasks unreliable, and similar problems can arise in stirred culture. These effects are perhaps similar to some of those discussed in Chapter 5, such as the long-term effects of incorrectly prepared inocula. It is evident that in these cases the genotype has been, in effect, distorted, and that normal biosynthesis is no longer possible. It is surprising that normality is so difficult to restore during further growth and replication. Evidently, restoration of the correct environment is too late to be effective.

6.3.4   The griseofulvin fermentation

The griseofulvin fermentation provides a useful example of the way in which a process was developed, and the way it was optimised to provide a balanced scheme. The first step was the establishment of a submerged production process (Rhodes *et al.*, 1957) and the isolation of mutants giving high yields (Aytoun & McWilliam, 1957). The main fermentation patent (Hockenhull, 1961) describes the optimal method of working and is interesting in that fermentations of over 400 h were contemplated. The patent is also interesting in the way it anticipates fermentations that are now developed and give maximum yields.

In this fermentation (Hockenhull, 1961) a corn-steep medium is used, with a sugar feed adjusted so as to hold the pH in the range 6.5–7.0. This adjustment is a matter of experience, since the feed-rate is altered before the pH changes occur; how to do this is known by practice. There is a good supply of nutrients at first, some of which soon disappear, such as the amino acids and ammonia.

70   *Submerged culture conditions*

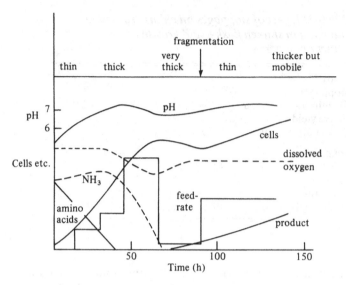

Fig. 6.2. Griseofulvin growth pattern.

Fig. 6.2 shows that a series of changes in the thickness of the culture took place as growth developed. Product formation started relatively late in this fermentation, at about 72 h. Before this occurred, the cell concentration rose steadily, in a form that gave a very thick culture, so thick that it would not pour from the sample bottle. Fairly soon after, and quite suddenly, by about 100 h, a marked change occurred due to fragmentation of the pellets. The culture became very mobile, remaining so even though it became rather thicker later. Owing to the thickening at 75 h, the dissolved oxygen started to fall, and this was relieved by the reduction of the feed-rate and by the thinning of the culture. Although rather dramatic, this picture is not unlike that shown by other fermentations. The penicillin Run 30 (Chapter 3.3) showed a sharp fall in dissolved oxygen at 24 h, relieved shortly after by a change in morphology and followed by a rise in dissolved oxygen which lasted for a considerable time.

These patterns show a continuous series of changes in cell conditions and medium composition. Once the culture settles down into the production phase, the steady state may last for many hours; with griseofulvin it may last for as long as 300 h or more.

The series of changes in the cells, the medium, and the environment, brought about by fragmentation, implies a series of changes in the phenotype. It is the complications produced by these effects that has led many workers to turn to continuous culture, where it is possible to hold the environment steady.

The graphs in Fig. 6.2 bring out a series of balances. In the first place the fragmentation of the cells enables the oxygen supply to be balanced against growth requirements. There is also the balance of sugar feed-rate against pH, which enables the fermentation to be held on the correct course and avoids a shift to an unfavourable metabolic pattern. There are also other balances connected with the disappearance of amino acids and ammonia, at an early stage, thus limiting growth during the production stage. It is known that the nitrogen level in the cells falls during the fermentation, suggesting that during the main production stage there is a dependence on reserves. There are probably other balances concerning phosphate and magnesium, which, under these conditions, will be mostly out of solution. Thus, the picture given in Fig. 6.2 means that a series of balances has been achieved, with all the important factors in griseofulvin production being optimised as a result. It is easy to see the control of sugar feed-rate by holding the pH steady as a simple control mechanism, while, in reality, it sets the cells into the correct mode for production and then maintains the process, which is really a rather complicated system.

To the modern reader, it is interesting that the measurement of dissolved oxygen, and oxygen transfer capacity, were not used in the development of the griseofulvin process. The fermentation process was seen as one that had to be operated within the capacity of the fermenter to sustain it, and the pH-controlled feed-process was used to achieve it. The fermenters used were undoubtedly efficient, and adequate for the purpose, in modern terms. The balance between the efficiency of the fermenter and medium and feed would be found by trial and error, backed up by experience in the way fermentations respond to conditions.

These results bring out the differences between genotype and environment. The genotype is stable, and responsive to conditions, while the environment is constantly varying during the fermentation, sometimes favourable, sometimes not. Balanced conditions in the environment, with respect to sugar supply, oxygen concentration, and cell condition, are necessary if production is to continue for a long production period. It is evident, from Fig. 6.2, that the changes in cell form are likely to facilitate rapid respiration and rapid growth, and that this is related to the agitation–aeration system in the fermenter.

6.4   Discussion

As revealed by the examples, the antibiotic production process is a variable and interactive system, involving the strain used, the medium, and the type of fermenter as it affects aeration and mixing. These factors interact in different ways, as shown by the way two mutants respond to conditions of stirring, the comprehensive changes in parameters produced by temperature, and the way a series of balances were achieved

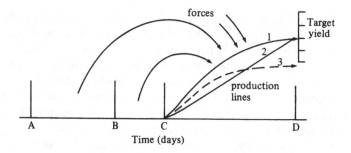

Important operational factors

Period	Important 'forces'
A–B Pre-production stage	Known to be important, and sensitive to error, in the start-up of penicillin, oxytetracycline, and griseofulvin. Length: 7–10 days.
B–C Start of production stage	Growth rate critical in penicillin and oxytetracycline. Length: penicillin, 0.5 days; oxytetracycline, 1.5 days; griseofulvin, 3 days
C–D Completion of production stage	Main effects of importance: growth rate, balance of nutrition to growth, oxygen supply, toxicity, enzyme stability. Sensitive to precursors, quality of materials etc., stoppages in agitation, mistakes in control. Length: 6–10 days

Fig. 6.3. Analysis and assessment of batch. A, start pre-production stages; B, start production batch; C, antibiotic production starts; D, end.

in the griseofulvin fermentation. The effect of the quality of the inoculum, and the later inhibitory effects that can arise, have already been discussed in earlier chapters. All these effects express continuous changes in the balance between genotype and environment, summarised in Equation 6.1.

Another view of these effects is given in Fig. 6.3. The diagram shows how each stage of the fermentation affects the end result by applying a 'force' to the production fermentation. The effect of these forces becomes apparent in the shape of the production curve, which may show different sorts of ideal production curves (1,2), or an inferior one (3) shown as a dashed line. The environmental forces acting on the fermentation may originate in any part of the fermentation. It will be realised that in a production batch the pre-production stages may require up to four steps and last for longer than the batch itself. At the earliest, the effects of these forces will begin to appear in the early stages of the batch itself, when they must be detected and action taken to ameliorate them.

To understand precisely how the positive and negative effects arise and work is difficult to define, but their existence as part of the way fermentations work has to be understood, and attempts must be made to define these effects and to design a fermentation programme that will provide the necessary balance and hold an optimal pathway. Similarly, a strain that is able to work well under diverse conditions should be much sought after, since it could lead to a stable fermentation (Young & Koplove, 1972). There will be further discussion of these matters in Chapter 13.

Part 2
Process development in the laboratory

Process development work involves two main areas.

(a) The discovery and isolation of microorganisms producing new antibiotics, as a result of screening programmes, and the development of efficient fermentation processes for the production of material for testing. This usually involves the production of improved mutants and media. The object is to provide material for testing, in the laboratory and clinically. To make larger quantities of material, pilot plant fermenters are often used.

(b) Development associated with manufacture; this may be simple at first, but of increasing sophistication as yields increase. Such work is usually done in research units at the factory.

The various classes of work to be done are: (1) the planning of fermentation experiments and the gathering of data, (2) the organisation and interpretation of data, strain improvement, and selection, and (3) development of processes that give maximised results, materially and economically, using techniques that become more critical as yields increase. These subjects form the bases of the chapters in this part of the book.

While academic work tends to be speculative, as it is intended to explore and expand scientific knowledge, industrial research may seem rather narrowly based. Industrial research requires very reliable experimental apparatus and results. For this reason equipment of a high standard is customary. In a recent article, the equipment for a pilot laboratory was quoted as costing £1.5 million, illustrating the degree of elaboration involved in this type of work. Such work is demanding and also very interesting in its own right for those who like to see a new discovery brought into use as an aid to humankind.

7 Laboratory fermentation process development

7.1 Introduction

The type of work required in this field is wide ranging and can vary from the simple to the elaborate types of experimentation. As experimental work is costly, there is a tendency to make many tests on individual batches, especially with stirred culture, and to obtain as much data as possible, often using standard routine methods. This can present a more-complicated picture than is currently needed, but it proves useful for future reference.

In earlier times, equipment was often designed and made by user firms. This was, in some ways, convenient, but it was expensive in time and in design costs. At present, equipment is usually made by specialised firms who supply not only shakers and fermenters but also ancillary equipment; these firms also carry out the installation. There is extensive instrumentation, both on the fermenters and in the analytical laboratory, and built-in computers are used for recording, control, storage of data, and its analysis. Some of these changes have been introduced to economise on staff and avoid over-night supervision.

To bring the subject into focus, Table 7.1 summarises some of the common types of fermentation apparatus and their intended uses. The numbers are not intended to be taken literally, but they give an indication of likely requirements. In general, the smaller sizes of equipment are used for academic work, or for screening and quick tests, where a few clear results are needed. Industrially, for laboratory work on process development, larger fermenters are preferred, for example 20–30-l capacity, so as to avoid confusion over volume changes and to provide for extraction work.

7.2 Apparatus for shaken culture

The general procedure used for shaken culture is described in Chapter 2.4. Spores are used to start an inoculum flask, and the resulting culture is added to production medium. Production cultures may be run for 4–14 days, and additions of nutrients may be made to prolong production.

The shaker involves three or four main parts. These are (1) a framework supporting the trays that hold the flasks in clips, (2) a support system that allows free but accurately controlled movement of the framework, (3) a drive mechanism that links the moving parts to the

77

Table 7.1. *Types of fermentation apparatus*

1. Shaken culture apparatus

Flasks	Size	Number of 500-ml flasks per shaker	Speed (rpm)	Use
Conical flasks	large	100–200		screening and
	small	10–20	200–500	development

2. Laboratory-pilot-plant equipment

Stirred fermenters	Size	Working volume (l)	Stirrer (diam.; rpm)	Use
	small	1–3	7–8 cm; 500–1000	research tests
	general	10–30	10–15 cm; 250–600	development and preparation
	large	500–2000	—	development and extraction

motor; this consists of gearing or a belt drive, and (4) the electric motor and speed control. The shaker must be well designed and well made if it is to give long, reliable service, year in and year out. This is particularly so currently, since there is a strong tendency to work at 500 rpm, as this gives conditions more akin to stirred culture. There is a risk when one of the older designs is changed to give the higher speed just by altering the gearing or the motor setting. The result is unreliability.

The firm of A. Kuhner, Basel, Switzerland, has been mentioned to the writer as making reliable high-speed shakers that are expected to run at 500 rpm for 5 years. There are no doubt others, but it is advisable to seek advice from shaker users on the matter. Regular servicing of shakers is essential, to avoid risk of breakdown and serious damage to the machine. A factor of importance, in many locations, is the availability of assistance from the maker or from a local agent, especially in obtaining spare parts. Experience has shown that brushless induction motors give the best service. Motors with brushes tend to wear out after a fair period of service. Shakers also tend to fail if working under dusty conditions. It is often advisable to have several smaller shakers instead of a single large one. This avoids sharing, a factor that can lead to stoppages when flasks are loaded and unloaded and includes the risk of someone forgetting to restart the machine. Stoppages are always harmful.

Accurate temperature control is needed. This means cooling, and good circulation of air to give an even temperature. These factors can be critical. Temperature rises to 30–35 °C have been experienced due to the absence of cooling, and this can have a serious effect. The temperature control problem also arises in small incubator-shakers. Frankly, the makers usually leave the purchaser to find out about this for himself.

The question of the rate of oxygen transfer is important. This involves two main steps: the passage of air into the flasks by diffusion, and the absorption of oxygen by the culture. As a rule, the flasks are plugged with cotton wool, but special commercial closures are available, which are said to give better diffusion into the flasks. In a simple form, one or two layers of lint or a filter paper might be used. To increase oxygen transfer to the culture, some workers use flasks that are baffled. These are made either by heating the side of the flasks and pressing in spikes or larger, wedge-shaped baffles, or by placing a spiral of stainless-steel wire (1.5 cm diameter) around the bottom. An example is given by Ghisalba, Traxler & Nüesch (1978). In the writer's experience, baffled flasks tend to produce foaming. For a description of shaken-culture methods, see Calam (1986).

7.3   Apparatus for stirred culture

Stirred fermentations tend to fall into two types: (1) fermentations designed to study a particular point, with a minimum of data collection, for example the testing of mutants or for doing preliminary work with new isolates, and (2) development fermentations, with the collection of large amounts of data. Even with the first type, data may be collected for future use.

7.3.1   *Fermenter apparatus*

Fig. 7.1 shows a small fermenter unit used at Liverpool Polytechnic for projects and research. It represents a common type of system used by students. On the right is a module that holds a 5-l glass jar fermenter, providing stirring, aeration, and temperature control. The fermenter is 15 cm in diameter. With a single multi-blade stirrer at 650 rpm it gives adequate mixing and oxygen transfer. Fermenters of this type are frequently referred to in the text. They are usually sterilised in an autoclave. This module will also hold a 14-l fermenter. In Fig. 7.1 the shelves in the centre carry supporting apparatus. At the bottom are analysers for carbon dioxide and oxygen. The module on the middle shelf contains meters and controllers for pH and for dissolved oxygen. It also provides two peristaltic pumps for addition of alkali or feed. The module at the top is an input–output unit that connects the apparatus to a micro-computer, seen on the left. This provides records by means of a printer, and it also provides control of the fermenter, feeds, and inputs.

This type of apparatus is convenient, but the small fermenter cover and its awkward situation limit the number of activities it can support. In industry the fermenters are usually larger and free standing, with bottom-entry stirrers and with entry ports both in the cover and at the bottom. They are sterilised *in situ*. This allows much greater flexibility in

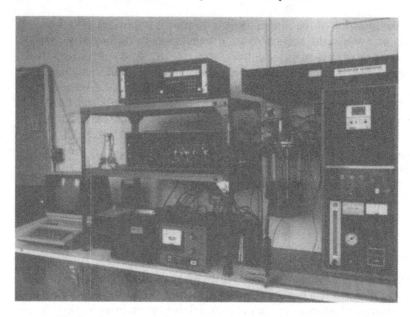

Fig. 7.1. Small research stirred-culture stirred-fermenter unit at Liverpool Polytechnic.

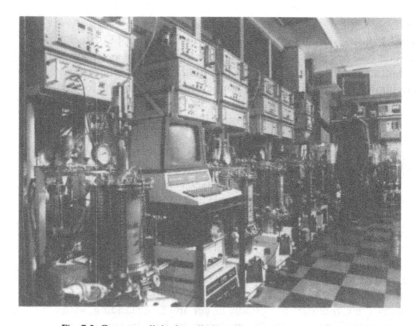

Fig. 7.2. Computer-linked small pilot plant fermenters in the Fermentation Development Department at Beecham Pharmaceuticals, Worthing, Sussex.

Table 7.2. *Fermenter equipment and supporting apparatus*

Fermenter fittings:
  Fermenter body; fermenter cover; agitator and baffles; bearings, gland, and drive; air-supply, inlet, air filter and outlet; sample line; entry points for instrument probes, feeds, etc.

Inputs and control:
  Temperature control; airflow meter; stirrer-speed control; pH electrode and controller, and alkali pump; nutrient feed inlet and calibrated pump; antifoam and/or vegetable oil addition system; oxygen electrode; output gas analyser (CO_2,O_2); other special systems

---

operation; also, with long fermentations, the replacement of instruments and of blocked feed-lines is readily possible. Such fermenters are usually assembled in pilot plants, as shown in Fig. 7.2.

With this type of modern equipment there are two main sections: the fermenter itself, and a cabinet that accommodates all the support equipment and the input–output connections to the computer. These can be seen in the background in Fig. 7.2. The system is largely computerised, and this includes the sterilisation process. For reasons of safety, the fermenters are made of stainless steel or suitably shrouded to avoid the risk of an explosion. The computer arrangements are often elaborate and are described later.

7.3.2 Auxiliary apparatus for fermenter operation

Table 7.2 gives a list of some of the main inputs and outputs involved in fermenter operation for monitoring, controlling, and feeding. As many as four or five feed-addition systems may be in use.

Essential equipment
Items in this category are the air supply, air filters, and flowmeter, the stirrer, and the temperature control system. A variety of air filters are used, the original type stuffed with cotton wool, and the newer sort consisting of a disc of filter material; both work well. It is important that the airflow is accurately measured, and flowmeters should be checked as the scaling may be approximate. The temperature control system requires both heating and cooling, and its operation must be checked from time to time. The stirrer is usually of the variable-speed type, and the speed should also be checked. The brushes in the motor should be regularly inspected.

Monitoring and supply equipment
pH. A pH-meter controller, with recorder, operates a small pump supplying acid or alkali, as required. It is convenient to use single-sided

control, using ammonia solution, which is also a nutrient. The quantity of
ammonia used is measured and is an indicator of growth.
Feed. A nutrient feed solution is often used so as to maintain a low level
of sugar in the medium. This is supplied by a pump, the rate being pre-set
or computer controlled. A second feed pump is used to supply vegetable
oil, which is a nutrient and also an antifoam.

Peristaltic pumps are used for these purposes. As large shots can cause
pulsing, which causes inefficient metabolism (Senior & Windass, 1980),
additions should be made as continuously as possible.
Antifoam. A sensor and small pump are used, though timed additions are
often satisfactory. The antifoam agents used may be polypropylene glycol
2500, or proprietary silicones. Care is needed with antifoam agents, as
they may appear in the product after extraction.

7.4   Analytical methods used in support of fermentation development

The following components are usually measured.
(a) Cell concentration.
(b) Culture volume.
(c) Product formation.
(d) Respiration: carbon dioxide produced, oxygen absorbed, and
     oxygen dissolved in the medium.
(e) pH level and pH-control requirements.
(f) Consumption of carbohydrates, nitrogen, and other nutrients.
(g) Minor constituents, e.g. NH_3, NO_3, PO_4, Mg, etc.
(h) Product toxicity.

Most of these analyses can be carried out by standard methods, usually by
automated methods, with the results being transferred directly to the
computer. Although analyses are expensive, a fermentation is a
multi-component system and can only be understood if a number of lines
of information are available. While the conversion and production of the
main components provides the main information, the relative rates of
disappearance or appearance of the other components may show
differences from standard patterns when fermentation conditions are
changed in experimental work.

As difficulties can arise in the estimation of the first four of these
components, a brief consideration will be given to them.

7.4.1   Cell concentration

Most workers find that the growth curve is an important factor in the
assessment of a fermentation. Unfortunately, the measurement of cell
concentration with complex media containing insoluble matter is not
easy. Filtration of a sample of the medium, followed by drying and
weighing, can give values of 5–100 g/l. After 24–48 h of fermentation,

80–90% of this may dissolve, and cell measurements may become meaningful, but there is always a degree of interference. In many cases, the growth curve has to be an estimate, as good as possible but not a precise measurement. It is often a model curve built around a number of data points, and examples of this procedure will be given.

The measurement of growth can be seen in two ways.

(a) As a scientific tool in research.

(b) As an indicator of the behaviour of the fermentation.

On the whole, in process development and plant work, the second aspect predominates. This means that quick and reproducible methods are needed for use as a basis for judgment in association with other data from the batch.

Cell concentration is commonly measured in four ways.

(a) Directly, by filtration of a sample (preferably weighed to allow for entrained air), followed by drying and weighing. Drying may be speeded by the use of an infrared lamp or microwave oven. Many antibiotics are insoluble at pH 6–7 and must be allowed for.

(b) Directly, as in (a), but including treatments to remove interfering substances, for example by shaking with a solvent to remove oil, or by acidification to remove calcium salts.

(c) By centrifuging and measuring the layer of cells, to give the packed cell volume (PCV) as a percentage of the sample volume. The cell layer can be removed, filtered, dried, and weighed.

(d) By indirect methods.

The subject has been discussed previously (Calam, 1969) and need not be expanded here. Indirect methods of estimation, e.g. from the nitrogen consumed, or from the content of protein, DNA, or ATP, are discussed in Chapter 13, and examples are included in the text. All these procedures depend on assumptions about cell behaviour and require a good practical understanding of the fermentation concerned. It is always important to be clear about the assumptions made, and about whether the results are sensible. Over-correction, to improve accuracy, can lead to results that may seem unreal in a practical situation.

7.4.2 Culture volume

In the course of a fermentation, volume changes can occur, which can give rise to confusion. A small fermenter, with 3 l of medium, can lose 125 ml by evaporation, at 25 °C, in 120 h. Removal of ten samples might remove 400 ml, or 300–400 ml of feed might be added, and water is also absorbed into the cells. These additions and subtractions, discussed in more detail in Chapter 11.3, could have significant effects on estimates of cells and materials; these effects are not easy to allow for convincingly. These effects are much less with larger fermenters (10–20 l); with these it is sufficient to give initial and final volumes of culture.

7.4.3   Product formation

Antibiotics may be measured directly against a test organism, or by chemical or physical means. The former, though less convenient, avoids the effect of similar but inactive materials. The use of high-pressure liquid chromatography (HPLC) provides specificity and is common practice. An electrode is available for the estimation of penicillin.

7.4.4   Dissolved oxygen and respiration

Dissolved oxygen can be measured with one of the commercial voltaic electrodes now available.

Carbon dioxide in the effluent gas can be measured with an infrared analyser, and oxygen can be measured with a paramagnetic instrument. Before reaching the analysers, the gas should be passed through a double-surface condenser to remove water, and dried with silica before reaching the oxygen analyser. The instruments are checked with standard gases. As a rule, the gas pressure is atmospheric; correction would be needed if the fermenter was working under pressure.

Instruments of the type desired are accurate to 1–2% of scale. This is adequate for the carbon dioxide analyser, with a scale of 0–5%. Since air contains 20.9% oxygen, the oxygen analyser must be scaled to 0–25%. An error of 1% would be quite significant, and would upset the calculation of the respiratory quotient (RQ). Industrial firms are now using mass spectrometers (VG Instruments, Crawley, Sussex) to provide more accurate data.

Oxygen and carbon dioxide can be measured accurately, in about 15 min, in a Haldane apparatus, but this is not convenient for routine use. Pocket analysers for carbon dioxide are available (Gallenkamp, London).

7.5   Collecting and checking results

The data obtained are of immediate and future interest, and it is important that they should be quickly stored and checked, to avoid loss of essential information. It is important to note: (1) the object of the experiment, thus explaining the incorporation of any special features, (2) the media and conditions used, (3) any accidental or other variations in the planned process, and (4) at intervals, the appearance of the culture, noting any significant changes. It is convenient to incorporate these details in the standard record form.

Results should be checked immediately for reliability, in case a technical fault has affected them. It is useful to quickly graph the results, for comparison with expectations, as this draws attention to any unexpected or missing information. Once the equipment has been switched off, it will be impossible to check any faults.

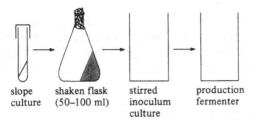

| slope culture | shaken flask (50–100 ml) | stirred inoculum culture | production fermenter |

Fig. 7.3. Steps in stirred culture.

In an experiment with a number of fermenters, statistical analysis is useful. Increased experimental errors are a sign of experimental faults. The analysts may be expected to have checked any results provided.

7.6 Steps in the operation of laboratory stirred fermenters
7.6.1 *Operational methods*

A brief, practical account will be given for those unfamiliar with the art. Shaken cultures are described in Chapter 2. Work in stirred culture is similar to shaken culture in principle, but the more-complicated apparatus and objectives present problems absent in shaken culture. The steps generally used are shown in Fig. 7.3. Stirred-culture inoculum is usually preferable to material grown in shaken flasks.

A slope is used to prepare a spore suspension, which is used to start a shaken flask culture. This provides a quantity of mycelial growth, which is used to start the main inoculum culture in a stirred fermenter. This may be tested by allowing a sample to stand, when the liquid should contain 85% or more of culture; alternatively, a centrifuged sample may be observed. As a rule, the best results are obtained if a stirred inoculum is used. The inoculum normally determines the performance of the production culture. The proportion of inoculum used is usually 5–10%.

After inoculation, growth commences quickly, accompanied by changes in appearance and colour as the batch proceeds. Sampling should be organised so as to obtain a number of points, which will facilitate the drawing of curves. At the end of the fermentation, it is advisable to take an extra sample, as this, if only 1 h after the 'final' one, is useful in confirming the final results.

The operation of successful stirred cultures involves many kinds of work, and experience is necessary to obtain the best results.

7.6.2 *Organisation of stirred-culture experiments*

The general methods for the operation of the fermenters will be found in the maker's manual. It is good to make some trials with water first to make sure all is well, and that the system is understood. During sterilisation, or if working under pressure, adequate safety precautions must be provided.

In setting up stirred fermentations, the handling of equipment and preparation of materials and ancillary equipment should be worked out with great care. It is best to have a written plan so that everything can be checked.

7.6.3   *Difficulties in fermentation experiments*

The main problems likely to arise are: (1) mechanical breakdowns in the apparatus, temperature control, etc.; any stoppage of aeration and stirring, for a few minutes, may be harmful, (2) failure of the culture to grow correctly and give satisfactory product yield, (3) foaming, and (4) infection of the culture with foreign microorganisms. The best defence against these problems is careful maintenance of the apparatus and anticipation of points where special attention is needed.

Beginners often find it difficult to make fermentations work successfully. It is not easy to overcome this problem. It may be easier to get started with shaken cultures, and to change to experiments with the more-complicated stirred culture apparatus later.

In the event of trouble, the best approach is to look at each step and ask the questions; Does it look likely to work? Does it work? If an unfortunate event has occurred ask: Why did it happen? Could it have been anticipated and avoided? What must be done to prevent it in future? For example, poor growth suggests that the spores or the inoculum were inadequate, or that the medium is incorrect. Tests can then be planned to test these things, probably in shaken flasks. If the process works in shaken flasks but not in stirred fermenters, then there must be something wrong with the fermenters. It may be that time has to be spent learning each stage of the process, even using simplified procedures and media. It is a matter of common sense. Obviously, experienced advice is a great help, and a visit to another laboratory could be the best way to solve the problems.

Foaming can be a problem. The cure depends partly on the choice of antifoam, and also on making additions to anticipate foaming, rather than waiting for it to start. Experience is often needed before foaming can be controlled. The type of strain and type of medium may be responsible.

Infection is often more troublesome in stirred cultures than in the simpler shaken cultures. Bacteria are the most common infectants, but yeasts can also give trouble. Especially during the early stages of development, all cultures should be tested by microscopy, or by adding 0.5 ml of culture to 100 ml of nutrient broth that is incubating, or by spreading culture on plates. Bottles or tubes should be incubated at 25 °C, as well as 37 °C, as many common water bacteria do not grow above 25 °C. The slopes and inoculum should also be tested.

With stirred fermenters, infection can arise because the fermenters are not fully sterilised. The usual sterilisation period, 20 min at 120 °C, may have to be increased to 30–45 min. The other main problem arises from leaks in the system. The equipment should be put under air pressure and leaks sought with soap and water. Faulty techniques may sometimes be detected by watching someone set up and start the process, to see if mistakes are being made accidentally.

These difficulties are usually cured by patience and careful observation. It is often helpful to change all routines, and the medium, so as to throw fresh light on the situation. The fact that reported fermentation programmes often start numbered in the twenties indicates the difficulties experienced.

7.7   Application of computer control in the laboratory
7.7.1   Types of computer systems

There is increasing interest in the use of computers with laboratory fermenters, as they can provide very flexible control over long periods; this control can be interactive with the fermentation conditions. Computers also keep clear, easily accessible records. Ryu & Humphrey (1973) described a number of pilot plant installations, and since then many papers have appeared in *Biotechnology and Bioengineering* associated with the work of Cooney, of Wang, and of others. There are many situations where a computer can help in development work, especially in providing 24-h cover for recording, with the addition of the application of intelligent control, derived from information being received from the instruments. Types of control used in research differ from those used in the plant; controls in the plant will be described later. At present, four main types of laboratory installations are in use.

(a) Small units, consisting of a cheap computer and interface, built up and programmed by the microbiologists concerned (e.g. Nelligan & Calam, 1983; Bu'Lock *et al.*, 1984; Vu-Trong & Gray, 1982*b*). Provided a suitable computer is chosen, having available 'add-ons' to provide an input–output system and amplifiers, this is not too difficult, but it requires skill and patience. On the other hand, the control program written will match the selected purpose. Systems of this sort are valuable for controlling and recording over long periods, with varying feeds and conditions, and are recommended for enterprising researchers. For guidance, the Computer Club of the Society for General Microbiology can provide help.

(b) Larger, chemical-engineering types of controllers have been described by a number of workers (e.g. Mou and Cooney, 1983*a,b*). They are elaborate and comprehensive, but less suited for microbiologists as the orientation is different.

(c) Small fermenters with associated computers are supplied by most makers. These are often programmed for control of pH and dissolved oxygen. In some cases machine code or a difficult language is used for the program, and accessing other instruments is not easy for amateurs of the art. It is advisable to find out exactly what is being provided. The system provided by Braun (Melsingen, Switzerland), programmed in BASIC, sounds suitable. These systems should be able to meet most requirements. Computer programs can usually be modified, but it often needs some skill and a degree of persistence.

(d) Large packages are available, giving multi-service monitoring over groups of fermenters, for example the Multi Fermenter Computer System (MFCS) of Ritenko of Finland. This can control each fermenter and give a quick presentation of its condition at any time. It accepts data from probes and from analysers in the analytical laboratory and passes the data, for storage, to the main computer. It can recall and present batch data in a variety of convenient ways. The system is too comprehensive to summarise, and it has great possibilities in the study of fermentations. It is a large computer package that can accept data, sort it into convenient forms, and then process it in a variety of ways, according to the needs of the operator.

A programme package of this type is ideal for the operation of a multi-fermenter, multi-user laboratory or pilot unit. It enables the users to receive first-class facilities for fermentation control, with an excellent record of results, which is permanently retained. The very clear presentation of results, in a variety of forms, and the avoidance of time wasting in data collection and calculation are valuable features. It also gives operators and users quick scans of the position in all fermenters, so that conditions can be readily checked.

Some workers find a system of this kind complex and rigid, intervening between the experimenter and the experiments. The question is whether efficient use of time and apparatus can be achieved in any other way. On the other hand, simple types of recording and pH control can be worked very well by analogue systems, often built into individual fermenter units. So much depends on the size of the development operation and the amount of information required from each experiment. If this amount of information is at all large, and the experimental system is elaborate, the computer seems the rational way ahead.

7.7.2   *Methods of computer control*

Four approaches to computer control can be observed, each of which covers a wide field of ideas. They may be summarised as follows.

(a) *Ad hoc* methods giving immediate control of behaviour.
(b) Anticipatory control.
(c) Adaptive control.
(d) Expert systems.

The great value of the computer is immediately obvious from this division. The computer is so flexible that the approach can be changed or modified as ideas change as to the best way to optimise a given fermentation. This gives an advantage over any electro–mechanical system. It is true that these approaches involve increasing theoretical and programming difficulties, but this should not prevent a move in a desired direction. At the same time, it must be said that everything still depends on the development of ideas and ways of using them; the mere involvement of a computer does not, in itself, help in this direction, except to provide a degree of freedom.

With fermenter units provided by manufacturers, computer facilities may not be adequate for dealing with subjects not thought of by the manufacturer. This can present a problem, but it can usually be overcome by a degree of determination.

In writing on this subject, it is necessary to introduce some material that will be discussed in more detail in later chapters, particularly in connection with plant control problems.

Ad hoc methods giving immediate control of batch behaviour
Typical applications here are the control of pH and of dissolved oxygen; these applications are already frequently used. Another application is the application of feeds, at different rates with time, according to the required 'profile'. The computer can also control routine additions of antifoam or precursors, on a time or demand basis. Many other applications exist, and these can often solve experimental difficulties and open the way to new ideas.

Anticipatory control
In the case of short fermentations (4–5 days), the process receives an initial impetus, which then dies away, giving a good yield of product. Production is really a one-phase matter, in which there is a single crop. Such fermentations need careful designing, but the factors involved are fairly simple. With longer fermentations (7–14 days) the cells have to be kept in an active state for a long time, and a more-elaborate basis for planning is needed, and a number of factors have to be taken into account.

Fig. 7.4 summarises the main factors involved in defining the behaviour of a production fermentation throughout its course; the figure shows three interacting areas. The first (1) is the fermentation itself, normally thought of as working ideally in accordance with its planned design, but it is strongly influenced by (2) the quality of the inoculum (Chapter 5) and by (3) the way the culture develops, in terms of thickness, oxygen transfer, and other ways.

In attempting optimal control based on microbial physiology, it is desirable to estimate the state of the culture, so as to anticipate changes, and to adapt the control system to suit the new conditions. For example,

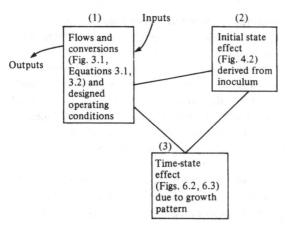

Fig. 7.4. Factors in determining fermentation behaviour.

if a feed is to be started or altered, the change must be made at the correct moment, and in balance with cell conditions. This is a situation familiar to process workers, who take anticipatory action on the basis of observation and long familiarity with the fermentation. This is the problem with *ad hoc* control. Usually it is successful, but if the response of the cells is not as expected, the resulting incorrect feeding can lead to poor results, or to pulsing and oscillation, which make the matter worse.

In planning anticipatory control, each antibiotic fermentation must be considered individually, in relation to the antibiotic concerned, the type of culture used, and the fermentation conditions chosen. Each fermentation therefore requires independent assessment.

Work on the penicillin fermentation has been reported by Nelligan & Calam (1983), who used a fed-batch process with a semi-synthetic medium. The fermentations were planned to consist of two stages: an initial growth stage, with $\mu = 0.06$ or 0.10, and a slower production stage, with $\mu = 0.010–0.012$. The effect of initial growth rate was shown by comparing the values of Y, p, and m in Equation 3.1 that are required to fit the growth data. For initial $\mu = 0.1, Y = 1.8, p = 0.21$, and $m = 0.014$; for $\mu = 0.06, Y = 2.5, p = 0.11$, and $m = 0.015$, showing markedly greater efficiency with slower growth. In this work, anticipatory control was obtained by measuring K_{La} directly and calculating the allowable oxygen transfer rate to maintain the dissolved oxygen tension (DOT) above 25%. This was compared with the planned transfer rate for oxygen, required by the calculated feed-rate, the lower value being chosen. This procedure was similar to that of Wang, Cooney & Wang (1979), and it gave good, smooth control of oxygen concentration. Further work in this field has been reported from Professor Cooney's laboratory at the Massachusetts Institute of Technology.

As an example of modern thinking, Mathers *et al.* (1986) have described the use of a computer-linked HPLC system to give feedback control based on the concentration of fermentation substrates.

Adaptive control
This is a form of control that has been developed as a general technique for use in control engineering. Work is now in progress on its application to fermentation work. It can be regarded as a more-advanced form of anticipatory control.

As generally used, data from the fermentation are compared, at intervals, with data from a model, and the state of the fermentation is recognised by the degree and type of fit. It is not essential to use a pre-set fermentation profile, because if a random feed is applied, the controller will re-set it. Adaptive control can be worked against a single factor, like dissolved oxygen concentration, or against several factors. The programmes used are complex but are based on standard routines that can be used on most large computers. But, for an understanding, a knowledge of mathematics is required. A useful example based on yeast growth has been provided by Yousefpour & Williams (1981). In Britain, work is in progress at the Polytechnics of Central London (Professor J. R. Leigh) and Liverpool (Dr D. Williams), and at the University of Newcastle (Dr G. A. Montague and Dr A. J. Morris). Publications have mainly been through conference reports, especially IFAC (International Federation of Automatic Control) and ICCAFT (International Conferences on Computer Automation of Fermentation Technology), but a number are in press in *Biotechnology and Bioengineering*.

This is an area of fermentation technology where much interesting work is being done, which is likely to increase in the next few years.

Expert systems
Over a number of years, computer programs have been under development which are capable of accepting information and using it to make decisions or diagnoses. These expert systems consist of a decision-making 'shell', in which can be inserted both quantitative and qualitative information, such as analytical results or estimates of colour shades. Programs can also accept 'don't know' responses. There is also space for the insertion of the rules used for the interpretation of the results. These rules are obtained from experts, since the formulation of them is often difficult.

Several expert systems have been used in medical work. A more-general example is the Savoir system (ISI Ltd, Redhill, Surrey), which has been used for counselling in agriculture; ISI Ltd also have other programs. In the system Expert Ease (Thorn EMI Software, Farnborough, Hants.), the responses of experts to sets of typical data can be inserted directly, the program making its own rules.

These programs can be run on bench-top computers. To an extent, the approach is the old one of consulting an expert, but the computer expert systems are not only more systematic, but also there when the expert is absent. They are therefore useful in the critical situations that can occur in fermentation plants, when consistency in decision making is of great importance. The incorporation of expert systems in methods of adaptive control is also under development.

7.8   Pilot plants

Pilot plants are intended to study fermentations, with a view to practical applications, and may be found in both research and works laboratories. They usually possess a number of fermenters of different sizes, often 12–20 or more, of 10–50-l capacity, and several with 1–4-m^3 capacity for extraction work. Pilot plants are operated by specialised workers, working on behalf of other scientists, and, because of their experience, they are able to produce maximal results. Typically, pilot plants are highly automated and computerised.

Fig. 7.2 shows a group of pilot plant fermenters of 10-l working capacity. It will be seen that they are computerised and provided with a full range of control systems. The figure shows up well the complexity of such systems and the expertise needed to operate them. It will be seen that this is essentially a working unit, applicable to a great variety of problems.

8   Assessment and understanding of experimental results

8.1   Introduction

At the end of a fermentation experiment, a set of results will be obtained. This may consist of antibiotic titres and some pH values, or, in a large-scale culture trial, there may be many results covering antibiotic production, growth, and other factors. An immediate requirement is to check the general appearance and behaviour of the culture to establish its normality and reliability. The analytical data can then be collected and examined.

As a rule, antibiotic production is a key indicator, while other factors express the manner of growth and metabolism. From these data it is possible to obtain a picture of how the fermentation works, and to obtain ideas for its future development.

It is possible to visualise the fermentation mechanism as like a wire sculpture, in which wires rise from the base, intertwine, and form a network tower. Here, the wires represent the reactions or material flows described in Chapters 3 and 4. One of these wires might represent growth, others might represent respiration and the use of nutrients and the behaviour of other reactions, but the most important one would represent antibiotic synthesis, which should ascend to the maximum possible height.

If the sculpture was based on theory, there would be many wires; in reality only a few reactions are monitored, so there would be only a few wires. These would represent factors that could be measured continuously, like pH, feed, carbon dioxide, and oxygen. But with growth and antibiotic production, measured at intervals, only beads would appear representing these spot values. In plant work, the sculpture might consist only of these beads. Evidently the linking up of these beads to form 'wires' is needed to produce a convincing model and facilitate its use. The object of this chapter is to consider how this could be done so as to obtain the maximum use of the available information, an essential step in experimental work. There is an obvious corollary, that the closer the beads are together, the easier it will be to link them together in a convincing way. Unfortunately, in industrial work, there may be gaps, and the use of complex media can cause bias in their location.

The assessment of the results involves three main areas, which provide the headings for the main sections in the chapter. These are: (1) the recording and presentation of the results, and, where necessary, the application of corrections, (2) the analysis and interpretation of the data, and (3) the visualisation of the patterns of behaviour in the fermentation, with a view to the interpretation of their significance.

8.2   The recording and presentation of data

8.2.1   *Appearance and morphology of culture*

It is generally felt, on the basis of experience, that there is a connection between the appearance of the culture (colour, thickness, texture, viscosity, pelleting) and its morphology (as seen with an optical or electron-scanning microscope) and its productivity. Righelato *et al.* (1968) have provided a study of one type of penicillin culture, and many other papers have appeared. The association between differentiation and secondary metabolism has been discussed previously (Chapter 3.4), and some results with *Streptomyces rimosus* are given in Chapter 3.5.

Although this is a difficult subject because of the complex manner in which microorganisms behave and because of the lack of a clear means of describing the changes that can be observed, there is no doubt that it is potentially of great importance. There are examples in the literature in which attention to culture morphology has been important in obtaining maximum yields. This is a subject that will be discussed later.

It is therefore advisable to examine cultures and make records of their morphology in submerged culture, especially in the course of mutation work, as an indication of changes in their behaviour, and to do this in such a way that the information can be recovered when required. This is also desirable as a means to detect culture degeneration, should it take place.

8.2.2   *Antibiotic production*

Assays of the antibiotic are usually made once or twice a day, preferably more often. With modern analytical methods, the test is likely to be specific and reliable. The results can be plotted on graph paper, and it is usually possible to draw a convincing curve. It would be better, however, to use a polynomial regression computer package, as this would be less likely to be biased and would indicate experimental error.

8.2.3   *The growth curve*

The establishment of the growth curve

Most workers find the growth curve of particular importance, as it expresses both the extent and the rate of growth during the batch. In industrial research, unfortunately, the use of complex media containing insoluble material can make it difficult to obtain useful data at first, and later only a few data points may be available. The problem is, therefore, to make the best use of the limited data to obtain the growth curve.

An immediate approach is to turn to data from work with synthetic media, so that practical growth curves can be obtained. With good inocula and well-designed synthetic media, rapid growth can be obtained, without any lag phase. This growth appears similar to that produced with complex media, at least in terms of the quantity of cells produced in a given time. From these data, model equations can be derived and these can be applied to industrial conditions, on the assumption that the same rules apply. Curves can, of course, be drawn by eye, but it is better to have a more rational basis of procedure. Provided good approximations can be obtained, which point the way ahead, it is better to move forward to new experiments than to spend too much time trying to obtain better accuracy. There are times when it is necessary to do this, but a more adventurous approach usually pays, provided mistakes can be avoided. It is a matter for careful judgement.

Fig. 8.1 shows a number of approaches to the problem. Two penicillin batches are considered: Run 9 with a semi-synthetic medium allowing good estimations of cell concentration, and Run 30, already discussed, in which insoluble material did not clear for some time, so that cell estimations were not possible until about 36 h. Growth curves were obtained by polynomial regression equations (using a computer package); from the carbon dioxide output using Equation 3.1; and using two growth-model equations, that of Yamashita, Hoshi & Inagaki (1969):

$$\mathrm{d}x/\mathrm{d}t = \mu_{\max} \cdot x \left(\frac{B - z \cdot x}{B + (\mathrm{J} - z) \cdot x} \right) \tag{8.1}$$

(where x = cell concentration (g/l), B = concentration of a limiting component in the medium, z = the proportion of B per gram of cells, and J is a constant), and the logistic law equation already described in Chapter 6.3 for penicillin modelling. In these fermentations, the initial concentration of cells was 1 g/l.

Fig. 8.1 shows that the polynomial equation gave a good curve for Run 9, where there was a good spread of data points, but with Run 30 the initial curvature was incorrect, there being no data for calculation. The carbon dioxide method gave good fits for both batches, as would be expected. The model equations worked well with Run 30, but the situation with Run 9 was more complicated, as the points suggested the occurrence of two growth phases. This was due to the use of two sugar-feed rates (Calam & Ismail, 1980), the rate being doubled at 55 h, thus allowing further growth. This effect could be overcome by using two sets of parameters for the equations, with a change at the appropriate time, so as to give good fits. With the logistic law equation, it was necessary to use a value for x_0 (concentration of cells at 0 h) of 3 g/l, to avoid an unrealistic growth pattern.

All four methods provide good possibilities for producing useful growth curves from minimal data. Of these, the carbon dioxide method is preferred, because carbon dioxide production is so closely connected

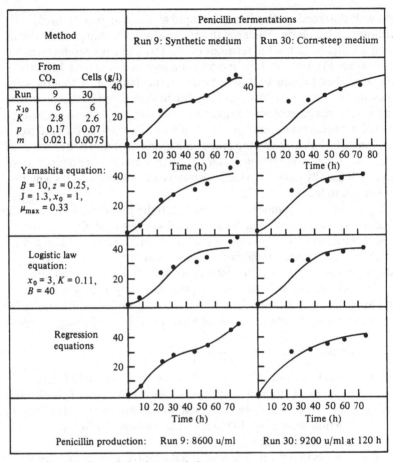

Fig. 8.1. Curve fitting for growth data.

with the growth process. In considering growth curves, it is important to keep in mind their fundamental shape, derived from the behaviour of microorganisms. This is stressed by the curves obtained with Run 9 and Run 30 by polynomial regressions. Both gave good fits, but one would be rejected as unlikely, because it did not fit the normal pattern of growth observed with these cultures.

Growth curves from batches with dense media
Situations can arise when only a very rough idea of the growth curve can be obtained, owing to the presence of large amounts of interfering material in the medium. The methods just described can then be used to produce as good a curve as possible, to help with the investigation of the fermentation. This is illustrated by a penicillin fermentation (Run 36, Calam & Ismail, 1980), in which the medium contained a large amount of

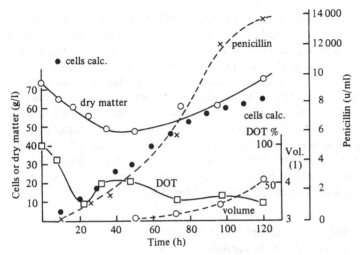

Fig. 8.2. Run 36: penicillin batch with peanut medium, corrected to 3 l volume. Parameters for estimation of growth from CO_2: $Y = 2.1, p = 0.1, m = 0.006$.

coarse peanut meal. Towards the end of the fermentation, most of the meal seemed to disappear, and some idea of the cell concentration could be obtained. Because the culture became very thick, water was pumped into the fermenter, increasing the volume from 3.0 to 4.1 l. To allow for this, measurements were corrected to 3 l, so that the final values reached artificially high values. The results of this experiment are shown in Fig. 8.2.

The growth curve was calculated from the carbon dioxide output, and it appears to be reasonable, under the circumstances. It will be noticed that the value for Y is lower than in Run 30, suggesting differences in metabolism, which were not unexpected.

A method such as this must obviously be used with caution. It can only give an approximate picture, and it is necessary to obtain as much evidence as possible to support the results obtained. The present work has been supported by trials with synthetic media (cf. Fig. 8.1) with both penicillin and yeast fermentations (Nelligan & Calam, 1980, 1983), which showed that this method could be used to predict cell concentrations with fair accuracy.

8.2.4   Importance of material balancing

The utility of this procedure as a check on the results has already been stressed in Chapter 3.3.

8.2.5   Degrees of freedom

The examples given in the text have described fermentations in terms of cell growth, product formation, production of carbon dioxide, dissolved oxygen, use of nutrients, and changes in pH. Thus an understanding of the fermentation is based on only 5–6 factors. From the point of view of statistical analysis, this would provide 4–5 degrees of freedom from which conclusions could be drawn. It is apparent that a fermentation is a multi-component system that involves many more factors than this. Experiments limited to this limited level of testing can therefore give only a limited picture of the system. Most of the experiments described here have been restricted in this way for the sake of simplicity. Simplicity has its virtues, but in serious work it is probably desirable to include more tests just to increase the area studied. This point is recognised by process development workers, who normally collect data upon a number of factors, thus increasing the degrees of freedom.

8.3   Analysis and interpretation of data
8.3.1   Analysis of data by the method of slices

Having collected and checked the data, the next step is to consider its meaning, with a view to finding key areas for investigation. As a quick approach, it is convenient to consider conditions and happenings at a series of points during the fermentation, noting changes in patterns of growth, conversion of material, respiration, production, and other factors. This can be done by considering 'slices' through the fermentation, and by taking 'snapshots' of the process at these intervals (Young & Koplove, 1972).

To illustrate this procedure, data was taken from Run 36 (Fig. 8.2). A series of six snapshots is shown in Table 8.1, covering a number of factors, which are often expressed as specific rates. As all these values have been corrected, they appear rather high. The actual final cell concentration was about equal to that in Run 30.

The snapshots show three main effects. Growth and production appeared to occur normally and smoothly, but it is clear that, in fact, the general metabolism became disturbed at about 80 h, when the pH unexpectedly fell and sporulation occurred. At 100 h there was a sharp fall in growth rate. The analysis shows unexpected events taking place, possibly due to a fall in DOT or to end-product inhibition. This suggests that while biosynthesis continued steadily until about 120 h, primary metabolism was collapsing and there was a shift in differentiation. This batch was expected to peak at 108–120 h, and this was achieved and could perhaps be improved a little by adjusting the medium. To make a major improvement, for instance to double production by 200 h, would require a much deeper investigation of the system, so that primary metabolism could be stabilised. Thus, the analysis by the method of slices emphasises the future more than the present.

Table 8.1. Snapshots: penicillin Run 36

Age (h)	20	40	60	80	100	120
Cells (x, calc.) (g/l)	10.9	27.2	40.3	55.2	63.9	68.2
dx/dt (g/l/h)	0.89	0.58	0.79	0.67	0.076	0.69
μ (g/g/h)	0.082	0.021	0.0196	0.012	0.0012	0.010
dCO_2/dt (l/l/h)	0.59	0.54	0.72	0.75	0.52	0.84
$(dCO_2/dt)/x$ (l/g/h)	0.054	0.020	0.018	0.014	0.008	0.012
dp/dt (u/ml/h)	70	90	110	130	200	80
Q_p (u/g/h)	6.4	3.3	2.7	2.35	3.1	1.2
$(dCO_2/dt)/(dx/dt)$	0.66	0.93	0.91	1.11	6.8	1.22
DOT (% sat.)	23	50	40	28	35	20
Residual lactose	36	15	trace	nil	nil	trace
Sporulation	–	–	–	+	+	+
pH	6.25	6.7	6.4	6.0(72 h)	7.0	6.9
4M NaOH added (ml, total)	–	–	0	10	60	175

Values corrected to 3.01. Actual concentrations of cells at 120 h, 50 g/l calculated, 56 g/l found. pH control from 76 h.

Table 8.2. Computer results from penicillin batch

Age (h)	50	75	100	132	142
% CO_2	1.09	1.14	1.59	1.96	1.75
CO_2 (l, total)	47.5	93.6	150.1	245.5	283
DOT (%)	82	77	42	43	41
K_{La}/min	10.3	7.4	3.4	4.1	4.0
dx/dt					
(total/h)	2.8	1.0	1.2	1.08	0.73
Glucose					
added (g)	93	181	276	472	525
Cells from					
CO_2 (g, total)	48.3	83.7	111.7	144	158
Volume (l)	3.3	3.6	3.9	4.35	4.49
Penicillin (u/ml)	1600	2800	5000	7200	8600

Airflow rate, 3.0 l/min.

8.3.2   On-line computer recording and assessment

The involvement of a computer in fermentation control and recording enables a large amount of data to be collected and snapshots of the fermentation to be obtained at frequent intervals. Table 8.2 provides a typical listing. It was obtained by the attachment of a computer to a small fermenter during experiments on the penicillin fermentation (Dr I. Nelligan, 1983, personal communication); the volume of culture was approximately 3.5 l, and the printed values refer to the whole culture. By modifying the computer program, automatic control could be applied; this was based on holding K_{La} above 4.0/min. The subject of the use of computers in fermentation work is a large one, and Table 8.2 gives an idea of the type of data that can be made readily available.

8.3.3   Computer modelling for co-ordination of results

Computer models can be of use in the study of fermentations since they allow a number of components of the system to be brought together. They can be used to analyse fermentation behaviour, or to predict the results of changes without the need for practical work. Models may be mathematical, or non-mathematical, with the concepts expressed by quite simple equations, which can be used together in a practical manner that is easily understood. These non-mathematical models are probably more suited to the microbiological mind, as are relatively unstructured computer programmes. Models of this kind can usually be expanded as required, but excessive expansion can lead to complications and the spending of much time with little result.

A simple, non-mathematical model is given in Table 8.3. It

Table 8.3. *Simple penicillin model*

```
    3   REM "run 30F"
   10   LET Pen=0: LET Qp=0: LET Dp=0
   20   LET X=1: LET Z=.25
   30   LET J=1.5
   35   LET Q=8.3: LET E=.02
   40   LET Y=2.5: LET p=.07
   50   LET n=.0075
   80   PRINT TAB 0;"T"; TAB 6;"x"; TAB 10;"Pen"; TAB 23;"co2"
   90   LPRINT TAB 0;"T"; TAB 6;"x"; TAB 12;"Pen"; TAB 23;"co2"
   95   FOR T=0 TO 120 STEP 2
  105   LET Pen=Pen + Dp
  108   IF T<51 THEN GO TO 125
  110   LET B=13: LET M=.16
  120   GO TO 130
  125   LET B=10.5: LET M=.30
  130   LET Dx=M*x*(B-Z*x)/(B+(J-Z)*x)
  136   LET Dx=Dx*2
  145   LET x=x+Dx
  155   LET x=INT (x*10+.5)/10
  160   LET dco2=(Dx/2)/Y+x*n+p
  250   LET Qp=Q*(EXP -(E*T))
  260   LET Dp=x*Qp*2
  290   LET dco2=INT (dco2*100+.5)/100
  295   LET Qp=INT(Qp*100+.5)/100
  296   LET w=T/10-INT (T/10)
  298   IF w>0 THEN GO TO 500
  299   IF T>0 THEN GO TO 305
  300   LET x=1
  305   PRINT TAB 0;T;TAB 6;x;TAB 12 INT(Pen);TAB 23;dco2
  315   LPRINT TAB 0;T;TAB 6;x;TAB 14;INT (Pen); TAB 23;doc2
  500   NEXT T
```

T	x	Pen	co2
0	1	0	0.19
10	6.1	193	0.43
20	16.2	811	0.61
30	25.3	1835	0.58
40	31.8	3014	0.52
50	35.9	4170	0.47
60	39.6	5226	0.5
70	42.2	6167	0.49
80	44.6	6987	0.49
90	46.3	7689	0.48
100	47.7	8283	0.48
110	48.7	8783	0.47
120	49.5	9200	0.47

incorporates three basic equations: Yamashita *et al.*'s (1961) equation for growth (Equation 8.1), Equation 3.1 to relate growth and production (with *n* instead of *m*), and, for penicillin, part of Shu's (1969) equation:

$$Q_p = Q \cdot (e^{-E \cdot T}) \qquad (8.2)$$

In this equation, Q is a maximum value for Q_p, E is a decay constant set here at 0.02, T is the age of the culture in hours, and e is the base of natural logarithms (2.718). The programme is iterative, with 2-h steps, printing every 10 h.

The parameters were adjusted to copy Run 30. As a feed was used, the parameter B (Equation 8.1) was increased from 60 h. Fig. 8.3 summarises the results, showing fits that are mainly good. It will be noted that this simple model took into account the three main flows, and that ten parameters were involved. Tests could be made with variations in these parameters and their effect on the relation between growth and productivity.

8.4   **Discussion**

The object of this chapter has been to discuss ways in which the value of data can be extended and coordinated by different types of equations and models. This is always important in development work, when fermentation facilities must be used to the full. When the position is rather unclear, there is always a tendency to spend time and effort seeking experimental clarification. In similar circumstances to this, during a discussion when a decision was needed, the president of an international corporation happened to be present. He commented that new investigations would simply mean delay, as the extra data would be unlikely to affect the decision to be made. Decisions on present data were needed. This is good advice in the present type of situation.

This chapter has been based on a few examples of fermentations and models. Fermentations chosen were those in which the data available were rather limited, to draw attention to the need for special methods. The equations and models are also unsophisticated and deal with only part of the carbon metabolism in the fermentations. Other workers would probably prefer different models and would wish to include other components, such as the nitrogen metabolism complex, sulphur, and perhaps inorganic constituents. It would be unmanageable to try to deal with these subjects here. These subjects will be found in the literature. The present model (Table 8.3) will be used again when considering approaches to fermentation development to maximum levels.

The analysis of the peanut-meal batch illustrates some of these points. The model makes it possible to derive a growth curve, and to carry out an analysis by the method of slices. Although this is speculative, the analysis shows that the fermentation ended due to a collapse of the system,

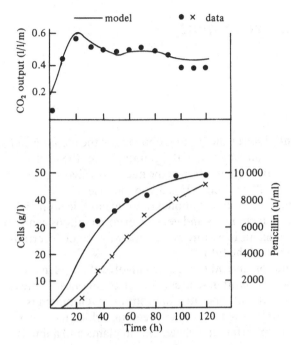

Fig. 8.3. Model of Run 30.

respiration becoming de-coupled from growth. The cause might be the fall in DOT, exhaustion of a major nutrient or of a minor one, or because of product inhibition. Model and data were insufficient to throw any light on these effects. This suggests that the next step is not to try to repeat the experiment on the old lines but with better growth data, but to investigate the factors causing this collapse, using new analytical and other methods, since the current ones are inadequate.

In development work, experiments are part of a sequence. Each batch is assessed during its course as well as at the end. There is no question of collecting data over 6 months and spending 3 months thinking it out. The use of computerised and automated systems cause results to arrive and require continuous attention. It is not always easy to adapt to this and to cope with the mental gap that can arise when a fermentation is a set of results and not a living thing that is almost a wild animal that has to be understood personally. In the old days, when streptomycetes were in use, you could tell how things were by the smell, detectable at the front door. This is a thing of the past. Not all workers find it easy to adapt to these aesthetic conditions. Adaptation to this situation, and the ability to visualise and use information, are part of the work of process development, which must be learnt and cultivated if success is to be achieved. Models are one of the tools that can be used in this connection.

9 Strain improvement

The productivity of antibiotic fermentations depends on the medium and conditions used, and also on the state of the genotype, i.e. the nucleus of the cells. Strain modification by mutation of the nucleus to give high yields has long been used and is illustrated in Fig. 3.9 in the case of oxytetracycline production. Mutation implies random modification of the nucleus. Recombination techniques and gene insertion methods can also be used to modify the nucleus in a more systematic way. Gene insertion appears to be the method of the future.

Since the use of mutation and other methods involve changes in the nucleus, strain development is often seen as a branch of genetics. There is no denying the connection, but, operationally, strain development is more akin to the long-established science of breeding, which has, over very many years, led to important improvements in plants and animals used in farming.

In strain development, the search is for new strains that (1) give better results and more product, (2) are capable of further development, i.e. have a flexible genome, and (3) are convenient in use. In breeding, the classical approach has been based on the careful choice of parental material, optimal conditions of culture for the expression of the desired effect, and detailed recording to aid selection and future planning. These points remain of maximum importance in industrial strain improvement. Selection is an important part of the system. Selection requires a great deal of work, and the choice of the correct system is of key importance.

Mutation produces both good and bad effects on the nucleus. Selection is usually only narrowly based, mainly on productivity. This can be harmful in the long term, since it can lead to improved strains in terms of production, but these strains can be difficult to handle and variable in behaviour, so that they become of little value. More-directed methods of improvement are therefore preferable, gene insertion seeming to have the most promise. Currently, expert opinion is that because of the complexity of antibiotic synthesis, which involves many genes, bioengineering is an alternative to mutation rather than a superior system. Judging by the great interest in genetic engineering shown by the manufacturing firms, it is highly likely that this will become a method of choice during the next few years. Such methods, relying on an understanding of biochemical systems and their regulation, require a much greater research commitment than does mutation, and mutation will continue to be of major importance, especially in the initial stages of strain development.

There are two outlooks on strain improvement. Geneticists are interested in nuclear behaviour and the question, how did this effect come about? This requires the use of biochemically marked strains so that questions can be answered. Industrial workers either are concerned with yield improvement, often using strains that have already been mutated many times before, or are concentrating on the quick mutation and selection of wild strains to give better results. They are therefore content to leave the questions unanswered. The descriptions here are based on this simple approach, which is usually sufficient for the advance to high or very high yields. Beyond this stage, problems may arise, which will be better discussed later.

Descriptions of mutation and selection work will be found in the literature, for example Calam (1964, 1970), Elander (1982), and many other papers. Rowlands & Normansell (1983) have written an excellent modern review, with many references. Convenient summaries will also be found in the reports on the 4-yearly Symposia on the Genetics of Industrial Microorganisms. Demain & Solomon (1986, pp. 154–215) provide an invaluable review, as do Vaněk & Hošťálek (1986, pp. 53–140). The latter contains a most valuable review of the work at Pan Labs on recent developments in the penicillin field, an area in which this firm has a leading position (Lein, 1986).

9.1   Methods of mutation

For this purpose it is usual to treat a suspension of spores, from fungi or streptomycetes, with a mutagen for an appropriate length of time. If the suspension is to be exposed to ultraviolet light, the suspension may be placed in an open petri dish and stirred with a bent glass rod, or suspensions in test tubes may be treated with chemicals. Mixed systems may also be used, for example a spore suspension may be exposed to ethylene imine and then to ultraviolet light, or spores exposed to ultraviolet light may be treated with caffeine to prevent re-activation by daylight. Slope cultures, preferably in thin plastic or glass tubes, may be exposed to gamma-rays or X-rays. Doses of 20 000–30 000 rads may be used.

Some of the principle mutagens used are the following.

(a) High-energy radiations: X-rays, gamma-rays, and fast neutrons may be used in the manner described above. If high-energy sources are used, exposures of 5–10 min will suffice.

(b) Ultraviolet rays: A suspension of spores is exposed in a shallow layer, as described above, under a bactericidal lamp, at a distance of about 10 cm, so as to give a kill of 90–99% or more. As described, treatment with chemicals may be used before or after exposure.

(c) Chemicals: A large number of substances are used. Those most commonly used are diethyl sulphate, ethane methyl sulphonate, and *N*-methyl-*N'*-nitro-*N*-nitrosoguanidine (NTG). Other chemicals are listed by Hopwood (1970). They are usually used at a strength of 0.05 M, with exposures of 5 min to 1 h, or as long as 12 h. The best lengths are only found by experience, as killing is often relatively low. A temperature of 25 °C should be used, as the effect is temperature sensitive. At the end of exposure, a few crystals of sodium thiosulphate are added to stop the action.

The radiations and some of the chemicals are potentially carcinogenic, and protective action must be taken to avoid risk of contact due to spillage or flying particles.

It is now generally recognised that particular types of mutagens have different effects on the nucleus. High-energy radiations cause breakages in the nucleus, while other mutagens affect individual DNA units. They therefore cannot be regarded as equal alternatives (Auerbach, 1976). When a series of mutations are being applied, the mutagen should be changed from time to time. In the writer's experience, the best results have usually been obtained with high levels of killing (99% or more) when using radiations. With chemicals, also, a high degree of treatment was preferred. Other workers prefer relatively low reaction levels. A judgement can only be made on the basis of practical results.

As an example of a mutation series, Heyes (1978) has described the improvement of neomycin production by *Streptomyces fradiae*. The wild strain gave 300 mg/l; this was increased by three stages of mutation with ultraviolet light followed by selection to 1000 mg/l. Two further stages with ethylene imine gave 1500 mg/l, raised by an X-ray mutation to 2000 mg/l. There were two other stages of selection without mutation, no doubt to purify and check the cultures. The best mutants resembled the parental strain; colour and morphological mutants were usually non-producers.

9.2   Handling, culturing, and preserving isolates

After mutation, the plating and culture of the colonies that develop is carried out in the usual way. The colonies are then counted and the numbers are compared with those from unmutated controls to obtain the percentage kill. The colonies can then be picked off onto slopes. Plating and isolation should be carefully planned, since only a limited number of colonies is likely to be needed, and a large number of unnecessary plates can be wasted. A method often used is to transfer whole colonies onto the slopes, which then grow out quickly, thus saving time. The slopes are examined after incubation. In general, the examination of the slopes is more useful than the examination of colonies on plates. Due to the proximity of other colonies, individual colonies do not always show the differences seen when they grow alone.

The slopes should be arranged in order of appearance and examined for colour, surface texture, colour of reverse, and pigment formation, according to the strain being used; undesirable forms should be rejected. Poorly growing forms usually do badly. Another undesirable point is the presence of mosaic effects. With these the colour or texture is not quite uniform but consists of tiny patches, varying slightly in colour. In other cases small sectors of different colour are detectable. These mosaic or variable strains may give high yields but are unreliable.

The slopes that are retained may be used for the first screen, but they are also sub-cultured onto several second-generation slopes. This stage of sub-culturing needs careful planning. The layout may involve:

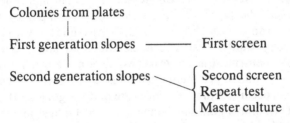

As a rule, it is desirable to put through each screening stage as quickly as possible, in a smooth operation, without having to wait to grow up cultures for re-test, as this would probably clash with other work. With careful planning, each stage may be completed in 3–4 weeks, ready for the next mutation.

When the results of the second screen appear, a selection can be made of potentially better strains. It may be necessary then to make confirmatory tests and to establish master cultures. As shown, allowance for this should be made when preparing the second-generation slopes, so as to avoid delay and confusion.

It is important to set aside and store a master culture of any potentially useful new strain. This means that a culture in good condition and ready for use will always be available when needed. Slopes of streptomycetes can be held at −70 °C. Fungi are more difficult, but storage is possible in liquid nitrogen, or spores can be held on silica. Small quantities of a solution of dried skimmed milk (5 g/l) are sterilised, as are 5-ml lots of pure, powdered, activated silica gel, in test tubes (sterilised at 150 °C for 2 h). The skimmed-milk solution is then used to make dense spore suspensions, 1 ml being added to a tube of silica (cooled in ice) and mixed well. The silica tubes can be held in closed vessels, dry, in the refrigerator.

Other storage methods can be used, but this method is convenient when large numbers are involved, many of which may be discarded. Important master cultures should be freeze-dried. The slopes should be briefly described, so that comparisons are possible later.

The writer's experience is that industrial strains are often subject to deterioration on prolonged storage unless great care is taken. Checks should be made at intervals. At all times it is advantageous to have spare master cultures of key strains, with a good description to enable full checking should this be necessary.

9.3   Methods of strain selection

9.3.1   Patterns of productivity in mutants and the use of preliminary screening tests

The result of the mutation is a number of isolates that should have a diverse range of production, compared with the original parental strain. Some of the new isolates should give increased yields. The main question is the ratio between the improvement in yield and the testing error. If this ratio is high, for example a doubling in yield, then a crude test with a high experimental error could be used for selection. If the advance was less, for example +25%, then a more accurate test would be needed. The example of the neomycin mutants, just mentioned, illustrates the changes in increase that can occur. At first, advances are quite large; later they are smaller, and it is mainly in this later stage when most industrial work is done. The situations described obviously differ from the selection of auxotrophic mutants, which differ totally from the parent strain and can be picked out by a very simple type of test.

A number of rough tests that can be used to detect mutants with a large increase in yield have been described. In most cases the mutants are plated and colonies are allowed to grow; then plugs of agar with individual colonies upon them are removed to an empty petri dish, and agar seeded with *Bacillus subtilis* or *Staphylococcus aureus* is poured around them. The plates are incubated at 37 °C and examined. Clear circles appear around the colonies; the diameters of these indicate the activity of the colonies (cf. Ball & McGonagle (1978), Normansell (1982)).

Consideration should also be given to growing mutants on small quantities of liquid medium in small cups in plastic blocks. This is followed by testing the activity using an automatic dilution and colourimetric assay system, preferably with computer recording, such as are available at the present time. Although strains may behave differently in surface and submerged culture, large increases in production would show up in this kind of test.

The potential usefulness of these types of tests is obvious, but critical reviews of their operation would be necessary from time to time, since the

Table 9.1. *Distribution of mutants in populations*

Quality of mutation	poor	standard	good
Frequency of improved mutants	1 in 40	1 in 20	1 in 10
Mean yield of improved mutants	+2.5%	+3.0%	+4.9%
Frequency of mutants improved by:			
5%	1/2000	1/200	1/50
10%	1/20 000	1/3000	1/300

effort involved would be wasted if they were rejecting good strains and selecting poor ones.

9.3.2 Selection with small advances in productivity

As yields increase, the best mutants will show advances of only 10–20% over the parental strain, and the advances may be as low as 5–10%. The standard error of single shake-flask tests has been found to be about ±10%, which is too high to reliably detect improvements of this level. If a population of mutants was tested, and the best one chosen and re-tested, the apparent high yield would be found to be due to error. Such a situation therefore requires a careful statistical examination to determine the best way to plan the screening system, so as to use the test facilities to the best advantage.

Such a statistical analysis was carried out by Professor O. L. Davies (1964), based on data from mutation screening programmes. This method, in different forms, has been used by a number of workers, with good results.

The investigation was based on computer studies. The analysis of mutation and testing data showed the existence of three typical populations, the characteristics of which are summarised in Table 9.1. The comparison of the observations shows the much higher frequency of mutants increased by 5%, compared with those increased by 10%. The frequency of mutants increased by 20% would be very much lower. It also shows the advantage of 'good' mutations, if they can be obtained.

On this basis it was possible to calculate the distribution curves, assuming a standard error of 10% for the standard distribution. The results of this are shown in Fig. 9.1. Graph a shows the expected curve, inclusive of experimental error. This is quite like a normal distribution curve, with a large proportion of mutants better than the control. Graph b shows the distribution without the error. It is now seen that nearly all the mutants are worse than the control, with only a small tail showing an improvement; it is mutants from this small group that are desired.

Using computer simulations, various schemes of selection were compared, taking into account the following considerations.

(a)

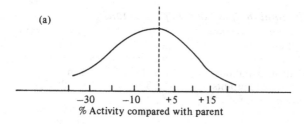

−30   −10   +5   +15
% Activity compared with parent

(b)

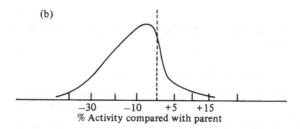

−30   −10   +5   +15
% Activity compared with parent

Fig. 9.1. Mutation: distribution of activity. (a) Including test error; (b) testing error eliminated.

(a) The distributions of mutants shown in Table 9.1.
(b) The standard error of a single shake-flask test at ±10%.
(c) That because small improvements are more common than large ones, yields would increase more rapidly by accumulating small mutations than by seeking large ones.
(d) That 200 flasks on the shakers were available continuously for the test programme.
(e) This implies that a continuous series of mutation cycles could be kept in progress. Instead of a single mutation with a test of 1000 isolates, there would be a series of mutations each with 200 isolates tested, thus completing 1000 tests in approximately the same time but with a much greater chance of encountering 'good' mutation steps.

The trials showed that two-step tests would be best. In the first step, 200 isolates would be tested with 1 flask each; in the second step, a proportion would be re-tested with several tests each with a greater degree of accuracy due to replication. Finally a few isolates from the second test would be kept. Examples of the systems investigated were:

Initial test	Second test	Retained
200 (1 flask each)	45 (4 flasks each)	10
200	32 (6 flasks each)	5
200	14 (14 flasks each)	1
200	50 (4 flasks each)	5

As a result of the statistical tests and practical trials, the last system was preferred.

It will be realised that a screen of this type does not identify the best mutant obtained; this is not the intention. It indicates that in the last five selected there are likely to be some mutants better than the parent, and others at least as good. The next stage is to mutate all five and test 40 isolates from each in the next cycle, i.e. 200 mutants. The best 40 of these are re-tested and five are retained, ready for the next cycle. After several cycles have been completed, it should become apparent that some of the selectants are better than the original strain, and these can be given supplementary tests. The system can then be reprogrammed. Alternatively, no progress may occur, and the position must be reassessed. It may be necessary to use a new starting culture, apply different mutagens, or introduce recombination techniques. Not infrequently, a programme may come to a halt, but progress begins again in further cycles.

If the standard system is successful, it will be found that advances often occur in a particular line of strains. The mutants selected at the end of the first round may be:

A   B   C   D   E

Then, after the second round:

A1   C1   C2   D1   E1

Then, after the third round:

C1.1   C1.2   C2.1   C2.2   D1.2

so that the line based on C is predominating. Experienced workers (Rowlands & Normansell, 1983) have pointed out the danger in this, because it may well be that the C-line of mutants may work well in shaken culture but fail in stirred culture or at plant level. It is therefore very important to include tests in stirred culture, as the programme progresses, to avoid waste of time with unsuitable mutants. This also stresses the importance of master cultures, so that a re-start can be made with mutants from more promising lines.

Mutation and selection programmes are normally continued for a long time. The programme needs to be constantly reviewed to make sure that there is a good opportunity for success. Care must be taken, as production increases, to make sure that the test method is adjusted to give optimal results. At higher production levels an increase in the supplies of specific materials in the medium may be necessary.

The system described depends on regular, short cycles of mutation and selection. This gives the maximum chance for efficient mutation to coincide with a strain responsive with the mutagenic effect. It has to be stressed that sensitivity to positive mutations varies greatly between strains, so that the inclusion of several strains, instead of only one, is an important feature of the system. It is advisable to vary the mutagens used.

The repeated cycles make it convenient to use overlapping systems, with two sets of mutants under investigation. This procedure allows a whole variety of ideas to be brought into use. The plan described is based on sound principles and well tested in practice, but it is also a starting point for development. Some examples of this will be mentioned later.

9.4   Alternative approaches to strain selection

The systematic approach just described has the advantage that it can be applied routinely with a good chance of success. Its use should not override the other possibilities, in which particular properties of the cultures being treated are made use of. This is particularly so when sensitivity to the product is a problem. It may be more important to increase resistance than to increase production alone. In such a case, mutation for resistance is an obvious line of approach. The antibiotic may not be very soluble in the medium, but there is a good chance that it will be absorbed by the cells, whether it is dissolved or not, if an excess is present, partly out of solution.

An interesting example of a mutation programme, strongly contrasting with the cyclic method just described, comes from Villax (1962), and it relates to the mutation of *Streptomyces albo-flavus*. A population of 3000 single-spore cultures was irradiated for 10 min/ day until sporulation occurred. Two single-spore cultures were selected due to their strong development and their very strong yellow fluorescence under ultraviolet light (Wood's glass). From these colonies, single-spore isolates were cultured and tested for production. The isolates showed a great variety of biochemical and morphological differences. The best isolate gave 7 g of oxytetracycline/l, which was 7–8 times the productivity of the parental strain.

This is an example of a mutation-selection programme based on a consideration of the special properties that were required in the strain being sought. Continuous reflection on the most appropriate approach to selection is always necessary and is stressed by Rowlands & Normansell (1983).

9.5   Recombination in strain development
9.5.1   *Methodology*

Most of the antibiotic-producing microorganisms multiply asexually, so that the full genetic mechanisms usually involved in hybridisation and crossing do not occur. Pontecorvo *et al.* (1953) described methods for achieving crosses in fungi by growing together biochemically deficient mutants, from which heterokaryons and, later, diploids arose. The diploids subsequently broke down into haploid recombinants, possessing characteristics derived from both parental strains. The mechanism involved was referred to as the parasexual process. It was later found that the same method could be applied to the streptomycetes. For a general account of these developments, see Sermonti (1969); later work is described in the various volumes arising from the Symposia on the Genetics of Industrial Microorganisms.

During recent years this approach has been greatly extended by the use of protoplasts. Early work with fungi is recorded by Peberdy & Gibson (1971; cf. Peberdy, 1979). Experiments with streptomycetes are described by Hopwood *et al.* (1977) and by Baltz (1978). Baltz (1978) fragmented biochemically deficient mutants of *Streptomyces fradiae*, and treated the fragments with lysozyme to remove the cell walls; this gave spherical protoplasts consisting of protoplasm contained only by the cytoplasmic membrane. Protoplasts from two strains were mixed and suspended in a medium containing polypropylene glycol 6000 and were streaked on agar, where normal-type colonies grew up, which were recombinants between the parental strains. Further work on protoplasts has continued extensively, for example Hopwood & Wright (1979, 1981). In the case of the streptomycetes, fertility plasmids also play a role in hybridisation techniques.

Reviewing the subject from the industrial point of view, Ball (1983) concluded that protoplast fusion appears to be a useful, cheap, and easy method to generate genetic variation in many areas of biotechnology. The impression given is that this is the method of first choice for this purpose.

The use of recombination techniques has been of great importance in genetics research. It has also been applied in attempts to increase production in industrial strains. This approach involves extra work both in preparing the mutants necessary for crossing, and in optimising the procedure, but its potential value in the interchange of genetic material is very great. However, attempts to use the method directly to increase production in fungi have generally been relatively unsuccessful, and the main advantageous possibility seems to be in the exchange of genetic material, which enables successful mutations to occur later. The general failure of crosses between high-yielding mutants to produce higher-yielding recombinants seems to be because the mutations to high yields in different lines seem to involve different enzyme systems that do not complement each other when crossed (Simpson & Caten, 1981).

In general, the greatest value of crossing procedures seems to be in the exchange of genetic material, which strengthens mutants weakened by prolonged mutation and selection, or by an increased sensitivity to positive mutations after crossing. These possibilities are discussed by Rowlands & Normansell (1983).

One aspect of crossing and recombination is that the results of individual crosses vary considerably in their effects, even when there is a common ancestry. These differences also show up during subsequent mutation and selection work. This is illustrated by an example from work on penicillin production.

9.5.2   *Example of recombination experiments with* P. chrysogenum

The application of recombination to penicillin production has been described by Calam, Daglish & McCann (1976). Diploidisations were carried out using biochemically deficient mutants from high-yielding industrial strains. In the first series, auxotrophic mutants yielding 6000 u/ml were obtained from parents giving 7500 u/ml of penicillin. The common ancestor gave 4400 u/ml. The object was to seek high-yielding mutants from diploids of these strains, and to consider whether the level of sporulation could be increased, since this had become reduced in the course of selection.

Ten diploids were isolated from the various crosses, with an average titre of 5500 u/ml. In the diploids, spore diameters were increased; in five cases this corresponded to a doubling of the volume. In five cases the increase in size was less, suggesting only partial diploidisation. The sporulation of the best diploids was five times that of the original haploid mutants. The diploids were mutated with nitrogen mustard (considered to be likely to cause minimum damage to the chromosomes), and 25 mutants from each were tested for penicillin production. Three cycles of mutation and selection were carried out in this way. The results in the best case are shown in Table 9.2. These mutants all gave very good growth and showed the compact form of surface growth associated with high-yielding strains.

The normal mutation programme was continued alongside these experiments. This involved four cycles of mutation and selection, giving a titre advance to 8500 u/ml, with continuing attenuated growth.

The best mutant from these trials was the diploid DC2/14 (ATCC46583). It has remained in use for laboratory work for 20 years, during which time there has been a slight loss of productivity. This shows that diploids are not necessarily unstable.

A number of sister-crosses were carried out, but these proved less promising than the original ones and did not show the expected hybrid vigour.

The results support those from other crosses with different fungal species (Calam, Daglish & Gaitskell, 1973). These show that diploids vary in their properties, and that to exploit the potentialities of the hybridisation technique, a number of crosses must be made, so as to find the best ones for future exploitation.

Table 9.2. *Results from mutation and selection experiment*

Diploid (u/ml)	Mutations (u/ml)			Spores compared with parent
	first	second	third	
4630	6780	6500	10350	×2

9.6 **Gene insertion and strain improvement**

The introduction of new methods in genetic research, whereby nuclei can be broken down and reassembled, with the introduction of foreign genes, has introduced new possibilities in the development of antibiotic fermentations. By the introduction of specific genes that confer improved biochemical efficiency, or resistance to the product, it should be possible to improve productivity in a specific manner that was not previously possible. Illustrations of this type of research are to be found in the work of Professor D. W. Hopwood and his team at the John Innes Institute at Norwich, where extensive investigations have been in progress for a number of years on the behaviour of *Streptomyces coelicolor* and other streptomycetes.

This approach to strain modification was opened by the discovery that genes conferring resistance to antibiotics can be transferred to infective bacteria by plasmids, and by discovery, later, that plasmid genes are involved in some types of antibiotic biosynthesis. At the second Symposium on the Genetics of Industrial Microorganisms in 1974, Collins (1976) described the possibility of gene multiplication by plasmid accumulation in the cells as a means of increasing biochemical activity, referring to work done with *E. coli*. This approach has been developed in many laboratories by extensive work on the modification, manipulation, and construction of novel plasmids. Around this an extensive literature has developed, only a fraction of which can be indicated here.

A general account of the methods used has been given by Old & Primrose (1983). It involves the following steps.

(a) Restriction enzymes (i.e. cellular enzymes that destroy foreign DNA) are used to cut up DNA strands from donor nuclei and from plasmids.

(b) Fragments are separated by electrophoresis and identified by specific methods. This process may be repeated, breaking up the fragments to give shorter lengths of DNA containing only a few or only a single gene.

(c) The fragments can then be reassembled to give new plasmids, which can then be cultured in a host bacterial population, on

which new properties are conferred. For the assembly of
fragments, ligases are used.

(d) Similar assembly of DNA fragments can also be carried out in
phages, which can act as vectors, but at present plasmids appear
to be preferred. An important feature of this type of work is that
a library of fragments can be set up, from which new phages or
plasmids can be assembled.

It will be appreciated that in the nucleus the order in which the genes
are arranged is of great importance. They must be placed in the correct
position in relation to promoter, regulator, and operator genes. Within
this general arrangement there are optimal patterns. It may be necessary
to construct a variety of plasmids to find the one most suited to
requirements.

Although the subject is in the area of advanced technology, the actual
techniques can be learned without too much difficulty, and the process of
gene insertion is regarded as well within the capacity of a well-organised
microbiological laboratory.

In applying the method to antibiotic production, the main problem is
our lack of knowledge of the precise nuclear changes that cause increases
in productivity. Even brief analyses of the position, either in biochemical
terms or on the basis of physiological parameters, such as have been given
earlier, show that a number of areas are involved, and that many genes
must be involved in the essential intermediate metabolism, while ten or
more genes must be involved in the biosynthesis itself. In the case of
oxytetracycline, Rhodes *et al.* (1981) have identified a considerable
number of genes. The manipulation of such a system is at present beyond
our means. It is still necessary to take a random approach, nowadays
referred to as the shotgun method. It is true that the important resistance
genes can be transferred, but whether this can give the high levels of
resistance likely to be needed in highly productive strains is not yet
known.

For these reasons, the main areas of progress in gene insertion have
been in connection with the production of hormones and other proteins
important in human physiology, of which insulin and the interferons may
be mentioned. In these cases, a single eukaryotic gene can be introduced
in a plasmid, which can then duplicate in *E. coli.* An example, illustrating
the production of human interferon, is provided by Vaks *et al.* (1984).
Although these methods have been very successful, and production in
stirred culture up to many litres in scale are taking place, there are still
difficulties, especially in the instability of some of the artificial plasmids.
Efforts are being applied to these problems, and, no doubt, solutions will
soon be found.

Another aspect of this research is the amount of detail of nuclear
structure that is being revealed. Gene mapping has become relatively

rapid, and fine structure is becoming more and more important when considering the design of new nuclei. In addition, many important pleiotropic effects are being revealed, not least the effect of new genes on the ability of the nucleus to mutate. The subject is still young, and many new developments are likely in the next few years.

9.7 Discussion

There is no doubt that the manipulation of the genotype is the main method of approach to high yields. Mutation and selection can carry output very far along the road to high yields, but the more directly genetic methods are more than useful supplements.

The methods used for mutation and selection may seem complicated, but once a system has been established, the technique becomes a rapid routine, capable of many modifications. Both of the genetic techniques, recombination and gene insertion, are claimed by workers to be straightforward. On the other hand, gene insertion must be more than a random process, and expertise must be developed or gained to facilitate the work. A great deal of commitment will be required for success. It is a subject for young, active, and adaptable minds with a capacity for seeing the order in complex systems.

It has been said earlier in the chapter that experts feel that antibiotic synthesis, which involves many genes, is a process too difficult to be dealt with at present. An examination of the results with oxytetracycline (Fig. 3.10), and of examples considered later, shows that maximum production involves primary metabolism and modes of growth, as much as, if not more than, sheer productivity, and that high resistance is paramount. The cloning of resistance is very much a practical proposition, for example in *Streptomyces rimosus* (Rhodes *et al.*, 1984), and other examples are quoted. The monthly British Patent Register for September 1984 showed nine patents in this field from Eli Lilly & Co., for example the cloning of resistance in *Streptomyces* species (British Patent 2,107,716). This suggests that whatever the difficulties the subject is in a rapid state of progress. As will be seen later, the achievement of maximum production involves many types of change in the mutants used, and the article by Lein (1986) is very revealing in this respect.

The present chapter has attempted to describe the situation as simply as possible, and it has been assumed that strains can be picked out on a relatively simple basis. In the later stages of development work, when strains are very active and the advances are small, considerable difficulties can arise. These will be discussed later.

10 Methods for laboratory process development

10.1 Introduction

10.1.1 The general problem

It is interesting to consider the problems that have to be solved in moving productivity towards high yields, based on a consideration of the material so far presented. While an increase in the specific productivity of the cells is important, many changes are also needed in primary metabolism and growth. Some of these are summarised in Tables 10.1 and 10.2. Table 10.1 lists some of the shifts in behaviour that are needed, while Table 10.2 shows some of the factors that have to be taken into account in both primary and secondary metabolism so as to obtain high yields.

Table 10.1 brings out the great differences between high-yielding and wild strains, especially the independence of secondary metabolism in relation to growth patterns and primary metabolism; the whole process of secondary metabolism becomes smoother and more flexible. Table 10.2 brings out the complexity of primary metabolism and the number of factors connected with it that have to be optimised to give good production. Secondary metabolism is, in comparison, simpler, though it depends on the properties of the cells being favourable to it. For the best results, secondary metabolism must be able to work well while primary metabolism is changing. Productivity is often connected to growth rate (μ). Productivity seems really to be related to the state of the cells. This may imply a particular value of μ, but cases arise where productivity is high, even in the absence of growth.

As mutation and selection take place, both good and bad effects are produced. It is possible that at some times primary metabolism may be optimal for production, and at other times it may be less good. The changes that may occur in primary metabolism may not be limiting at first, so that production continues to increase. Later the effect may become apparent. The fact that OTC⁻ mutants could no longer be recognised by a modern identification procedure (Al-Jawadi, Wellington & Calam, 1985) is indicative of the variety of changes in the genome that can arise when mutations aimed at increasing secondary metabolism are involved.

These observations show that process improvement is complex. It is possible to ignore this for a long time, as usually happens with early successful working. As time goes on, however, it becomes necessary to take some of these effects into account, in a more detailed manner (cf. Lein, 1986).

A feature of development work is the importance of working at

Table 10.1. *Pattern changes needed in process development*

Factors	In wild strain	Needed in high-yielder
Metabolism	restricted	smoother
Morphological differentiation in submerged culture	obviously stepped	smoother and simplified; adaptable
Link between primary and secondary metabolism	close	independent

maximum levels of productivity, at the expense of scientific clarity. An important aspect of this is that in production work, fermentations must be driven so that they proceed on an optimal course. While in the initial stages of testing, conditions may be based on experience, but it soon becomes necessary to lay down a carefully planned system of operation. New mutants and processes must be tested using the optimal, driven conditions. More relaxed tests, giving greater clarity due to the simplified conditions, can help at some stages of the work, but they can be misleading since the patterns of intermediate metabolism may well be different.

Because of the different conditions in which the strains work, from wild strains to high-yielding mutants, the subject of development will be considered in three stages, corresponding to the differing situations and objectives likely to be encountered.

Table 10.2. *Some important factors in high-yielding cultures*

In primary metabolism	In secondary metabolism
Adaptable genotype	Specific productivity (Q_p)
Inoculum and fermentation conditions	Resistance
Differentiation	High daily production increment
Cell concentration. Growth rates and respiration Dissolved oxygen	Enzyme system stability
Pellet type and viscosity	
Cell biochemistry, regulation, and physiology	

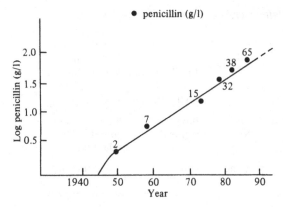

Fig. 10.1. Increases in the production of penicillin.

10.1.2   Rates of improvement

It is important to have some indication of the likely rate of progress in mutation and selection programmes. Fig. 10.1 gives a plot of some penicillin data, based on different sources of information.

The main points are the early, fairly rapid rise in production, after which there seems to have been a doubling every 6–7 years. It is thought that other antibiotic fermentations have behaved in a similar manner. Patience is evidently needed.

The graph must be interpreted with discretion, because up to about 1960, fermentations were fairly short, 4–5 days; since then the fermentations have gradually lengthened to 12 or more days (cf. Fig. 3.9d). Thus the advantage in product concentration and economic yield have not gone entirely hand in hand.

Continuing the subject of rates of progress, Table 10.3 shows levels of production of different antibiotics in 1969, based on figures given to an expert committee. Although these figures are historic, they do give an idea of progress made in certain lengths of time. The value for penicillin is roughly in line with that shown in Fig. 10.1.

10.2   Stages in process development work

In the field of antibiotic production, several phases of development work can be identified. These are summarised in Table 10.4, referring back to the concepts expressed in Table 1.1.

Each field involves its own types of problem and methods of working, some of which have already been discussed. Each field is likely to take a number of years, and with a new process, it takes many years before the

Table 10.3. *Antibiotic production levels
in 1969, after 15–20 years*

Antibiotic	Date of discovery	g/l in 1969
Penicillin G	1929	9
Erythromycin	1952	3–4
Oxytetracycline	1949	12–16
Chlortetracycline	1948	12–16
Streptomycin	1944	10
Neomycin	1949	8

Based on I. Horvath (1969, personal
communication).

Table 10.4. *Fields in process development: tasks and problems (overall
time-span, 20–40 years)*

Stage and objective	Type of development work	Limits to be overcome
(1) To give 1–2 g/l	development of new isolates, producing new antibiotics, to provide for initial tests	the organism's metabolic pattern that holds back production
(2) To give 5–15 g/l	increasing yields to high or very high levels for industrial production	the interaction between the needs of the organism and the ability of the fermenter to meet them
(3) To give 25–75 g/l or more	to maximise industrial production and economics	new techniques must be devised, and new strains developed, to remove the limits in stage 2

third stage is reached. A worker in process development may find herself or himself very much wrapped in the problems and techniques of a particular stage, which are naturally very detailed. It is only possible, here, to touch on some of the main points, without dealing with the many day-to-day problems of each stage of the work.

10.3   The initial development stage

This subject was recently reviewed by Richtie (1985), and his lecture will be used as a basis for a description of the work likely to be required. New isolates are obtained as a result of screening programmes, which start from the isolation of colonies from soil or other materials (cf. Chapter 2.1.2). The isolates are then identified, and selected strains are tested using specialised and mechanised methods aimed at the detection of substances having special types of activity. The principles used in these screening procedures have been described by Nolan (1986) and by Demain & Solomon (1986, pp. 24–31). In screening, the isolates are grown on several media, and the test results give a basis for choosing conditions for experiments on the production of the antibiotic concerned.

When promising strains are obtained, they are grown in shaken-flask culture (Chapter 2.4.2) using a variety of media, and tests are also made in stirred fermenters. On this basis, small amounts of product can be obtained for preliminary tests. If these tests show promise, an initial process improvement is started to facilitate the further stages of the programme, when large amounts of material become necessary. These quantities of material would be difficult to obtain if the original isolate gave only a very low yield, and this work could excessively monopolise the department's equipment. Most laboratories engaged in this type of work have pilot-plant fermenters of 0.5–2.5 − m^3 capacity that are used for this purpose.

Table 10.5 summarises the steps envisaged by Dr Richtie, in this stage of development, and also gives the sort of time likely to be involved. It will be seen that there is plenty of time for development to proceed.

It will be appreciated that 2500 l of culture, containing 0.01 g of antibiotic/l would give only 12.5 g, at 50% extraction efficiency. A tenfold improvement would give a clear advantage.

On this basis, Dr Richtie recommended the start of mutation and selection at an early stage, the multi-line approach being preferred. Yields up to 0.5–1.0 g/l could then be obtained. He stressed the importance of plating producer strains, and the selecting of cultures that were stable on sub-culture. He also stressed the need to have a well worked-out plan for dealing with potentially valuable isolates, to ensure rapid testing and exploitation. The failure of a culture to achieve the hoped for level of activity should not be allowed to lead to a gap in the

Table 10.5. *Initial development of new isolates*

Step	Objective	Quantity required	Conc. in medium	Time (years)
1	Isolation of new strains and preliminary test	1 g	0.05–0.15 [a]	1–2
2	Initial animal test for activity and toxicity	10–50 g		
3	Long term tests in animals, in 3 stages	(1) 3 kg (2) 35 kg (3) 50 kg	1	5–7
4	Clinical tests	500 kg	1–2	—

[a]Minimal yields may be as low as 0.005 g/l.

programme while new plans were made. A programme of this type involves a great deal of expertise and investment finance. The management of such a programme, involving other departments of technology, also requires a great deal of skill and patience, among all concerned. It is not always realised that the learning of these management skills has to be actively and positively learned if success is to be obtained.

10.4 Process development at higher production levels

When a strain has been isolated and improved so as to give a useful product at a level sufficient for the initial testing stage, development moves onwards to the achievement of higher production levels. In Fig. 3.9 this corresponds to parts b and c.

Many of the types of work involved have already been described. The main ones are mutation or genetic treatments, followed by selection, along with modifications to the fermentation so as to increase its efficiency. Summarising this work, the stages in each cycle of optimisation are presented in Fig. 10.2; The basis is scientific opportunism, that is to say, tests are made and possibilities for increases are noted and developed, there being, as yet, insufficient information for a systematic analysis of the problem.

An example of this type of scientific opportunism was the introduction of the lactose + corn-steep liquor medium for penicillin production. This was mainly based on experience rather than direct evidence, and led to wide-spread advances. In another case, a product was formed on a medium containing a large amount of sugar. From a consideration of costs, a trial was made with starch; a few flasks used wheat flour as something even cheaper. There was a significant increase in yield, but the

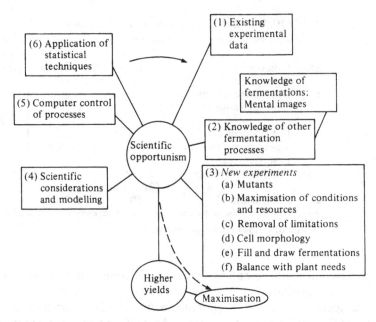

Fig. 10.2. Aspects of process development: cycle of considerations.

main effect with the flour was halving the production time. This again led to further developments. In cases like this it is possible, afterwards, to understand the cause of the effect and to exploit it in a scientific way, but the initial step is essentially opportunistic.

At this early stage, insufficient information will prevent the identification of the precise route to progress, and observation points the way ahead. The stages in the cycle develop the early indications and provide the subjects for the sections in this chapter. It will be realised that this stage of development work will probably occupy a number of years, and that stepwise increases will be made. During this time the cycle will be re-surveyed, and on each occasion specific areas will receive attention.

In industrial work, relatively short-term targets are set (e.g. 1 year). It is always wise to have targets, as they provide times when the work can be re-assessed and modified. Often a number of lines are in progress simultaneously, and much experience becomes available, which gives a basis for better assessments of problems and possibilities.

It will be realised that here it is only possible to review these aspects of development very briefly. In the laboratory each stage of analysis would require a considerable amount of reading and research before the next step could be approached.

10.4.1   Study of local information

The quality and extent of the work done in the initial stage of development can vary considerably, from fairly elementary experiments to enable production, to carefully developed and monitored trials.

Some of the main criteria involved in successful process operation have already been outlined in Chapter 1.1. The present section envisages a study to establish whether the initial process was reliable, and whether the mutant was good enough to form a basis for new work. The use of an unreliable process can lead to many difficulties and delays. It might be necessary to put in a good deal of work before a new campaign aimed at high yields could begin successfully. In any case, an inadequate basis might not provide evidence that could be used for forward planning.

In some cases it is very difficult for a considerable time to obtain high yields, and for initial manufacture it is necessary to accept a medium level of production rather than a high level.

The assessments considered at this stage form the basis for planning the work described in stage 3 in Fig. 10.2.

10.4.2   Literature information on fermentation processes

Although process development work relies mainly on practical trials and investigations, it is highly desirable to have a basis of theories and ideas, and to be aware of the outlook of other workers who are expert in the production of a range of antibiotics. A few examples are listed here, based on work in which high levels of production have been described. These should lead into the appropriate literature, where more detail is available.

Penicillin

Penicillin is usually made with complex media, frequently containing cotton-seed meal (cf. Beechham Group Ltd, 1968; Queener & Swartz, 1979; König, Schügerl & Seewald, 1982). Owing to the presence of nitrogen and sulphur in penicillin, and the need to supply precursor, the supply of all these materials is critical. Phenylacetic acid, added as a precursor, is used as a carbon source, thus raising a complication, and phenoxyacetic acid is preferable; this gives a different penicillin, not suitable for every purpose.

The biosynthesis of penicillin is known to start with the formation of a tripeptide, aminoadipoyl–cysteinyl–valine, from aminoadipic acid, cysteine, and valine. The peptide is subsequently cyclised and the aminoadipic side chain is exchanged for a suitable precursor, such as phenylacetic acid, but the mechanism involved in the formation of the cyclic nucleus remains unknown (Roberts, 1984). Two major biochemical effects that have been observed are the effect of the precursor in determining the type of penicillin formed and in stimulating the synthesis of nuclear material, and feedback inhibition of biosynthesis by lysine (Demain, 1957) and by penicillin itself (Martin *et al.*, 1979). Addition to the medium of the two main precursors, cysteine and valine, tends to inhibit biosynthesis (Roberts, 1984), but the side-chain precursor (e.g. phenylacetic acid) stimulates the synthesis of the central ring system. The usual sulphur source for the biosynthesis of cysteine is sulphate; the conversion requires much energy.

Hosler & Johnson (1953) developed a fed-batch fermentation using a continuous feed of glucose and a synthetic medium and giving yields as good as with corn-steep media. Many workers have used this process in research, e.g. Mou & Cooney (1983*a*,*b*), and Nelligan & Calam (1983), and this has led to much interesting discussion (Queener & Swartz, 1979). As might be expected, a good supply of oxygen, a resistant culture, and good inocula are needed, and the initial rate of growth during the production stage is also important.

Cephalosporin C
Cephalosporin C, another β-lactam antibiotic, is produced by *Cephalosporium acremonium*. During biosynthesis, the same tripeptide is formed as with penicillin, but the subsequent cyclisations are modified, and the aminoadipic acid side chain remains in place.

Fermentation conditions are rather similar to those with penicillin, but methionine is added to increase production. It was originally added as a potential source of sulphur. The synthesis of cysteine occurs by a single route with penicillin, but by alternative routes with cephalosporin C, the second route being suppressed by methionine (Drew & Demain, 1975). Methionine is also important because it induces the formation of atherospores in the mycelium, which are required for maximum production of cephalosporin C, i.e. methionine is an enhancer of differentiation.

In an interesting paper, Huber & Tietz (1983) have investigated the production of cephalosporin C using a fed-batch process with synthetic medium. Their paper is of particular interest because a high-yielding, commercial mutant was used. The media used for the preparation of inocula are interesting in showing the types of complex media used commercially; they are based on molasses, fish meal, peanut meal, calcium hydroxide, methionine, and lard oil. The authors note that when the secondary inoculum medium is used for production, the RQ indicated that lipid was being oxidised and the sugar was not used.

The initial defined medium contained glucose, ammonium chloride, methyl oleate, and metallic salts, and a feed of glucose was provided. This gave growth but little cephalosporin C. Production of cephalosporin C was induced by addition of methionine, which caused the necessary thickening of the mycelium and raised cephalosporin C production to about 4 g/l. There was a further increase if the glucose was added as a feed instead of at the start. Further experiments showed that if the feed of glucose was replaced by a feed of soya oil, so that a steady concentration of 20 g/l lipid was maintained, production of cephalosporin C increased to 12 g/l in 120 h. During production, growth continued steadily. The use of a feed of oil also gave a more easily controlled fermentation. A fermentation system of this kind obviously forms an excellent basis for research investigation. Several further examples of cephalosporin C production are given by Küenzi & Auden (1983).

Tylosin
Tylosin, discovered in 1961, is produced by two strains of *Streptomyces fradiae*, NRRL 2702 and 2703. Later (French Patent 1,497,830) it was reported that in shaken flask culture, with a medium containing fish meal, beet molasses, soya oil, $CaCO_3$. $(NH_4)_2SO_4$, and NaCl, NRRL 2702 gave tylosin at a yield of approximately 4 g/l, increased to 6 g/l by addition of a very small amount of hydrolysed tylosin, which evidently stimulated the fermentation process. Tylosin is a macrolide. It is known that in the fermentation several related compounds are produced alongside tylosin, of which macrosin and relomycin are the most important.

During investigations at the University of New South Wales, the production of tylosin was studied using synthetic media. Gray & Bhuwapathanapun (1980) studied synthetic media based on glucose, sodium glutamate, methyl oleate, and metal salts. Batch fermentations showed a growth phase, followed by a stationary phase during which tylosin was produced to the extent of 1 g/l, accompanied by the formation of the related compounds. Continuous culture work followed, with different ratios of glucose and glutamate. Glutamate appeared to reduce the specific uptake rate of glucose and increased the specific production rate of tylosin (Q_T) 3.7 times. By careful adjustment of conditions, tylosin production was obtained while growth was continuing.

The metabolic regulation of tylosin production was further studied, in continuous culture, by Vu-Trong & Gray (1982*a*). The principal enzymes in the synthesis of tylosin are methylmalonyl-coenzyme-A carboxylase and propionyl-coenzyme-A carboxylase. These reached maximum specific activities after 72–96 h of fermentation, while macrosin $3' - O$-methyl transferase (converting macrosin to tylosin) also peaked at that time and correlated with the maximum value for Q_T. The specific rate of tylosin synthesis was inversely proportional to μ and to the intracellular level of the adenylate pool, which seems to be associated with tylosin production.

Further work (Vu-Trong & Gray, 1982*b*) demonstrated the stimulatory effect of feeding glutamate and glucose at regular intervals of 10 h, glutamate for 0.5 h and glucose for 0.25 h. This had the effect of breaking up the repressive effect of glucose and preventing its effect on synthesis. This allowed tylosin production to occur during the initial growth phase as well as during the later, slower phase of growth. This cyclic feeding system increased tylosin production to 1.5 g/l in 240 h. It was considered that much of the advantage of complex media may be due to the different rates at which nutrients become available over successive periods. Much of the increase in production was due to the conversion of relomycin to tylosin.

Chlortetracycline
Extensive work on the metabolism and regulation of *Streptomyces aureofaciens* during the production of chlortetracycline has been done at the Institute of Microbiology in Prague, mostly using a semi-synthetic medium. A paper by Hošťálek & Vaněk (1973) gives a useful review and opens the way into a whole series of interesting reports on different aspects of this well-known fermentation.

Gibberellic acid
Attention is drawn to a very interesting account of the development of this fermentation, by Vass & Jefferys (1979). It involved the growth of the organism, and then a careful system of feeding which held the metabolic system in a balanced state, so that gibberellic acid was formed over a long period, with the formation of a minimum of fat. Fat formation is a normal last stage with this fermentation, gibberellic acid being produced for a relatively short period of time.

Oxytetracycline
The development of this fermentation has already been discussed, and the data is presented in Fig. 3.9. An initial mutation step increased specific productivity (Q_{OTC}) and lengthened the production period. Further mutation doubled production (Fig. 3.9c) almost entirely by extending the production period. All the evidence shows that the strains were strongly inhibited by the product.

Discussion
The examples above are all based on work with synthetic or semi-synthetic media. This may seem to be a distraction when the main weight of practical development is based on complex media, which may be cheaper and more reliable. Additionally the biochemistry and physiology of the fermentations in synthetic media may be significantly different. None the less, these investigations can be of great value to the investigator, especially if the yield of antibiotic is comparable with that with complex media. There is first the design of the synthetic-medium

process, which usually involves a feed. This design brings out the framework of material flows needed to produce good results, and the biochemical balances involved. The essential features, like the use of vegetable oil or glutamic acid as principal nutrients, stress the entry of major components into central metabolism by a 'side entry' as being important, as brought out in Fig. 4.1.

This practical analysis of the system, especially of the factors that determine optimal growth and production, is free from the makeshifts that are necessary with complex media. This analysis and new opportunities for analytical and microscopical studies of the culture also help towards clarity and encourage speculation and thought about the way the culture develops and reacts during the process. This is helped by continuous computer recording of respiration, accompanied by conversion to key parameters. With complex media, it is possible to see from the data that 'something has happened'; with synthetic media there is a better chance of finding out what it was. Clarification of this sort leads into and encourages biochemical studies. At the end of it all, the problem will remain complex and solutions may be partial, but new perspectives and concepts, produced by examining an alternative type of fermentation process, are almost certain to pay off in future.

In general, it can be said about the examples that they show much in common, but each involves individualistic details that make them unique. It is a problem for a development worker to think about his or her own different product and to hold together aspects similar to other antibiotic fermentations, while keeping the necessarily individualistic view that the particular case requires. The problem is to maintain the right balance. This can only be done by reading, thinking, and discussing, and gaining the necessary experience. The writer, having worked for a long time with antibiotics, became involved with a commercial anaerobic fermentation. It was surprising to find how well its behaviour fitted in with previous experience. All this is part of the process of learning, which is important in development work, and of forming mental images of fermentations and their mechanisms. These images can be used as points of reference in problem solving and planning.

10.4.3   Starting new experimental work
General
A number of headings are given in Fig. 10.2 to suggest areas of work likely to be involved; the order is not significant, and mutation implies any suitable method of genetic modification. This subject is easier to discuss in a practical situation, when information is likely to be available and it is easier to be realistic.

The amount of work to be done is usually large, and several lines will be investigated at once. It is possible to pick out a number of key ideas for initial investigation; these ideas will identify obstacles to development and give priorities for study.

The first step is to consider the potentialities of the existing process, and the particular problems to be overcome. This usually involves trials of media and conditions to see if production can be increased directly, and metabolic studies to discover the factors that determine the yield. The use of optimal conditions, giving the highest yields, brings out the major factors involved, especially product inhibition. Results obtained under sub-optimal conditions can be misleading, though they are sometimes helpful in bringing out important details.

General process improvement involves testing different media under different conditions. It is not always easy to invent novel media, and it is convenient to accumulate a small library of media, from the literature, containing the media and conditions used by other expert workers. These can be used as a basis for trials. The *Journal of Antibiotics* seems to contain many examples, and some of the references given here will help. It is also useful to collect a number of growth and production curves for different high-yielding fermentations; these are useful for comparisons.

Many initial experiments will be carried out in shaken flasks. It is good to bear in mind that future requirements will be for work in stirred fermenters, small or large, so that it is best to use fast shakers, giving high aeration and mixing, to obtain a degree of compatibility.

Establishment of growth and production patterns
An initial step is to carry out some stirred fermentations and observe the relation between growth and production. To these should be added some measurements of respiration and dissolved oxygen. Even if a total analytical scheme cannot be adopted, a number of spot measurements of carbon dioxide, done with a pocket meter (Gallenkamp, London), would be useful. Changes in pH should also be noted, as excessive variations from neutrality are harmful and require control. The morphology of the cultures should be given attention, as distortion or autolysis of the hyphae suggest death or damage to the culture.

As mentioned previously, the measurement of cell concentration can be difficult with complex media, but, at least, packed cell volumes can be obtained. If the layer of cells can be separated, it can be removed, dried, and weighed to give an estimate of the cells and to supply a multiplication factor. Even if an accurate curve cannot be obtained, it is useful to know the approximate cell concentration during the production phase (see Chapter 8.1).

One of the key values is the maximum specific production rate ($Q_{p,max}$), since it is possible to derive from it the maximum degree of production possible. Supposing that, in a fermentation lasting 120 h, the main production phase of 50 h has an average Q_p of 2.5 mg antibiotic/g cells/h (with a maximum of 4.0), and the cell concentration is 25 g/l; then the total production will be 3.1 g/l, probably plus a little more formed during the declining phase of production. This immediately raises the question of why the cell concentration is so low, and the production phase is so short. With the cells at 35 g/l and a production phase of 80 h, the yield would be 7 g/l.

Methods of analysing the situation have been given earlier and could be applied here. The three likely possibilities are: growth restriction due to shortage of nutrients; overloading of the oxygen supply (indicated by low levels of dissolved oxygen); or the development of toxins or inhibitors in the medium. These toxins would also reduce production. The first of these could be investigated by balancing and by analyses, the second by tests with increased oxygen supply. In stirred culture this could be done by increasing aeration or the rate of stirring, or by addition of oxygen to the air supply, so as to keep up an adequate level of dissolved oxygen without alteration of the other conditions.

The question of toxicity is more difficult. A simple test would be to centrifuge a quantity of culture aseptically, add some nutrients, and re-inoculate to see if growth occurred. In work on spore production by *Penicillium chrysogenum* (Frank, Calam & Gregory, 1948), inhibition of growth was found to occur. The metabolism solution could also be supplemented and solidified with agar and poured into plates. These could then be spread with normal or mutated spores to look for resistant strains which could be further developed.

The ideas suggested here are only a few of those that would arise in an investigation as new clues were revealed both by the experimental work and by the literature.

Extension of production by dilution and withdrawal
It has been found that production can sometimes be caused to continue if growth can be caused to continue at above a critical minimum rate. Dilution can make this possible, while holding the cell concentration at a constant level. This system can be used to enable the fermenter to be filled up to more than the normal level, or further quantities of culture can be obtained by withdrawal of part of the culture for extraction. An example of this is given in Run 36 (Chapter 8.2). A further possibility is the repeated withdrawal of culture, with subsequent re-filling and feeding, so as to give a series of culture increments. This substantially increases production from an extended batch and avoids the cost of restarting new batches. It therefore provides a novel approach to a substantial increase in production, with possible economies.

For such a system to be successful it is necessary that the culture is stable. This is not always the case. Run 36 gave a good yield up to 120 h; some culture was then removed and replaced with water, but there was no further production of penicillin, due to the collapse of the fermentation system (Chapter 8.3). With synthetic medium, however, and the same strain of *P. chrysogenum* and the same conditions, the culture proved stable. In an experiment, the initial 3-l culture was fed and diluted; four lots of 0.5 l were removed; and the batch was finally allowed to increase to 4.17 l. Penicillin production in the fermenter was 32.9 mega-units, plus 10 mega-units in the removed material. Other workers have obtained similar results.

Speaking at a meeting in Dijon, France in 1974 (unpublished), Professor A. E. Humphrey elaborated a method, using this method. After the culture had grown for 75 h, a 20% portion was replaced with salts solution, feeding being continued. At intervals of 40 h, four more withdrawals and additions were made, so timed to avoid dissolved oxygen falling too low due to increasing viscosity. The system was controlled by computer to give optimal conditions. Double the normal volume of culture was produced, in less than double the time, giving an economical process.

Although the proposal attracted a good deal of interest, it is not well favoured industrially. Objections are the extra nutrients needed to grow the replacement cells and the loss of nutrients during withdrawals. Although the extra volume gives more product, the titre is lower, leading to inefficiency in extraction. The discharge of the culture to an unsterile collection vessel (if only indirectly) would also produce a serious risk of infection.

During this stage of development, cell morphology in stirred culture tends to become more favourable to mixing and aeration, as a result of the general selection process. This can be critical, an aspect of the subject that will be discussed later.

10.4.4 *Scientific considerations and modelling*

Having obtained the new experimental data, it is necessary to consider them scientifically to seek new leads and plan trials. This has to be done against the background of a general knowledge of microbial behaviour, such as has been outlined in the earlier part of this book. The precise directions that these considerations will take will be determined by the nature of the fermentation under study, and it is not worthwhile to speculate on the matter in a general way.

Modelling is a useful tool in this situation, since in a model a number of ideas can be brought together and their interactions can be investigated. Table 8.3 has presented a simple model whose properties were explained, and this will be referred to again later. It is always best to keep models as simple and comprehensible as possible, as it is easy to waste time on elaborating them.

In preparing a model, the various components that one wishes to incorporate should be brought together; these components may include growth, production, consumption of oxygen and sugar, K_{La}, and the like. These can then be expressed by simple relationships at given intervals (e.g. 5 or 10 h) during the fermentation. As with Table 8.3, equations can be used to produce the curves. It is also possible to insert the proposed values as data, which are then read during each cycle of computation, producing the desired interactions. Other relationships, such as that between cell concentration and K_{La}, can be obtained from experimental data. A model formed in this way can be checked against experimental data and then used to test other experimental patterns in a most useful way. It can indicate whether proposed experiments are likely to be useful or not and help in understanding possibilities and planning experiments. If the model fails to predict results correctly, then it means that one's understanding of the system is incorrect. This simple approach is often better than waiting while a powerful model is produced; the powerful model may arrive too late to be of use, but discarding it may not be politic.

10.4.5   The use of statistical designs in experimental work

When research is in progress, many factors have to be taken into account. Therefore experimental planning becomes very important because of the demands such complex systems make on experimental facilities. This is especially so with stirred culture, because the number available is usually limited. The best possible use has to be made of small groups. The optimisation of a typical system might easily involve four or five factors, such as spore concentration in the inoculum, the age of the inoculum, the production medium and the feed pattern, the speed of stirring, and other things. Four factors at three 'levels' would require $3 \times 3 \times 3 \times 3 = 81$ tests, or five factors at two levels would require $2 \times 2 \times 2 \times 2 \times 2 = 32$ tests. If only four to six fermenters were available, and each test took 10 days, such a programme would be intolerably long. The use of statistically designed experiments, using fractional replication, or an optimal pathway approach could greatly reduce these numbers by giving brief tests. The results obtained from these could then point to further experiments.

The use of statistical methods is often disliked by microbiologists, who see statistics as a mysterious and inconvenient mathematical process that simply tells you that your results are not significant and the whole thing must be done again. This is too pessimistic. Correctly used, statistical methods can help design the most economical experiments and maximise the information available for a given amount of work. An expert has commented that experienced development workers do not need statistics to tell them whether the results are significant or not; what they want from statistics is to know whether the planned experiment is worth doing, and what to do if it is not. In this way effort is saved.

The involvement of statistical design means less fermentation work, but more time spent on calculation. Reduced experimental work, with a limited number of fermenters or shaken flasks per experiment, means scope for a much wider approach, and it is therefore worthwhile spending time on calculations, so as to produce more information.

Two useful experimental designs

The methods to be discussed here are the use of fractional factorial designs, and the optimisation methods of Box & Wilson (1951), which give the quickest pathway to the optimum. As previously discussed, experiments with four or five factors require a large number of tests. These numbers can be reduced by doing a fraction of the total, for example with three 'levels' of each component, by doing one third, or with two levels, by doing one half, one quarter, or one eighth. An alternative is the use of fractional Graeco–Roman square systems, described by Küenzi & Auden (1983).

The advantage of fractional replication is to use a smaller number of tests to give a good idea of the main results, so as to free time and effort for other investigations. The results of the original fractional test can always be confirmed by a second test, re-designed in the light of the information gained. This method has long been used in agriculture, where it may be possible to do only one test per year, or in the chemical industry, where individual tests may be time consuming and expensive.

A large number of fractional replication schemes have been worked out. An alternative is for a worker to select a few combinations from the total, and test those only. This tends to leave large areas of possibilities unexplored, and to reduce the accuracy obtained by replication.

To illustrate the arrangement, a simple $2 \times 2 \times 2 \times 2$ experiment will be described, using a half-replicate design. This experiment concerned the effect of four factors on the production of spores by *Penicillium notatum* on agar medium, with or without peptone, with or without addition of ammonium salts, with either sucrose or molasses, or with glycerol or acetate in the medium. The spores were grown on agar in large bottles, and suspensions were made from these. The reduction in design saved a great deal of labour. The resulting spore counts are shown in Table 10.6. The design was one used in agricultural research. For each main factor, four results were averaged. As the addition of ammonia had no effect, the table could be re-written without it, giving a normal $2 \times 2 \times 2$ design.

This simple experiment illustrates a technique of great practical use;

Table 10.6. *Spore production, half-replicate experiment*

		Spore concentrations ($\times 10^6$ ml)			
		glycerol		acetate	
Factors		sucrose	molasses	sucrose	molasses
Ammonia −	Peptone −	—	4	1	—
	Peptone +	121	—	—	68
Ammonia +	Peptone −	4			11
	Peptone +	—	166	17	—

Averaged main effects ($\times 10^6$/ml)

Sucrose	36	Ammonia −	49
Molasses	62	Ammonia +	49
Peptone −	5	Glycerol	74
Peptone +	93	Acetate	24

Based on data from Frank *et al.* (1948).

details of this technique can be found in the literature (Davies, 1967). Another approach to fractional designs is given by Küenzi & Auden (1983), who emphasise the way in which this system quickly weeds out factors that can be ignored and stresses those that need to be followed up.

The other statistical technique mentioned, developed by Box & Wilson (1951), uses a series of small experiments. The results of these experiments point to conditions giving an increased yield and lead to a new small experiment giving further guidance. The technique ends with a definitive test locating the maximum. Assuming that a number of factors are involved, these can be regarded as producing a multi-dimensional structure, which can be expressed as a mountain whose height is shown by contour lines. Such an arrangement is shown in Fig. 10.3a. The first set of tests might be centred on a point A, the results pointing to a second location B. Around point B, a new, small experiment can be designed, giving a pointer to C, near the summit. A final test would be needed to locate the best conditions. It is an unfortunate fact that often there is no clear peak (Fig. 10.3b), and the ascent is to a plateau (Calam & Russell, 1973). If the plateau is located, the reason for its existence can be examined. It is clear that there is no point in proceeding as if a summit existed.

The mathematics involved are too complex to be explained here, but they could be handled by a suitable computer package. The Box-Wilson method is described by Davis (1967), and its applications to antibiotic fermentations are described by Auden *et al.* (1967). See also Demain & Solomon (1986, pp. 41–8).

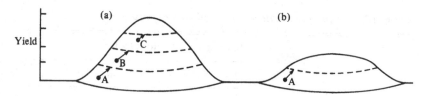

Fig. 10.3. Optimisation by steepest ascent.

10.5   Antibiotic production at maximum levels

10.5.1   Introduction

The production of very high antibiotic titres (15–20 g/l, in the terms used in this book) has been described in the previous section as a result of scientific opportunism. Culture conditions were modified on the basis of experience. The typical types of growth and production curves obtained are illustrated by Queener & Swartz (1979) and here in Figs. 3.9c and 8.3. Rapid growth occurs at first and gradually slows down; the production curve is rather similar but commences after a lag of a day or two. The high vitality of the cells gradually fades, and biosynthetic enzymes decay; the end of production is likely to be due to cell death, enzyme decay, the onset of product toxicity, or limitations in the oxygen transport system. Even if resistance to the products was increased, oxygen lack would end production as the cell population exceeded the biological space available. As the snapshots in Table 8.1 show, a reconsideration of the whole fermentation is necessary; this will result in different patterns of behaviour throughout the process. This is already foreshadowed in Fig. 3.9d. It marks a change in the original opportunist approach, to one that is systematically based on a study of the fermentation system.

This systematic approach began to appear in the 1960s, typified perhaps by the griseofulvin process (Hockenhull, 1961) and in an account of developments in penicillin production (Hockenhull & McKenzie, 1968). These processes were probably indicative of industrial development, generally. They were characterised by long production periods (up to 400 h with griseofulvin) with limited growth. Although yields were high or very high, and did not approach current maximum levels, the fermentation pattern was already moving in the desired direction.

The change is indicated in Fig. 10.4, which shows the flows of materials in high- and maximum-yielding fermentations. With high-yielding processes, the flow (Route 1) is into primary metabolism, with an overflow into secondary metabolism, while with maximum production the route only minimally involves primary metabolism.

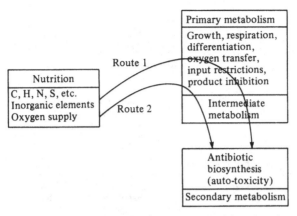

Fig. 10.4. Areas and routes in metabolism with high and maximum yields.

The carbon balance for a penicillin fermentation that gives about 6.5 g of product/l, is shown in Table 3.2. Of 65.6 g carbon input to the system, 3 g passed to penicillin, while the energy required for synthesis would take a further 7 g (assuming 2.2 l of oxygen/g, and RQ = 1). With a batch giving 65 g of penicillin/l, over 100 g extra carbon might have to be input, 30 g going to penicillin, and 70 g for energy. This is bound to require a re-routing, as in Route 2, where much of the nutrients pass to intermediate metabolism, for biosynthesis, very little going to primary metabolism. Under these conditions, growth will be minimal, though the TCA cycle must be very active so as to supply energy for maintenance as well as antibiotic synthesis.

In ordinary fermenters, the cell concentration is brought up to its upper limit, so the yield cannot be increased simply by growing more cells. It is known that with maximum-yield batches, growth is deliberately limited by the availability of inorganic elements, especially phosphate. This will also have an effect on metabolic routing.

The implication is that a new pattern of growth and production will be needed, so as to give stable production for a long time, and the growth form must be such as to allow good oxygen transfer. In the absence of detailed information, it will only be possible to discuss this in a speculative manner, but sufficient information is available to obtain useful clues as to the methods used.

An analysis of the problems involved is attempted in Fig. 10.5, in which the several layers involved are presented in three shells. The first of these (Shell 1) summarises the main fermentation process, as already described. All of these are linked to the need for process stability (Young & Koplove, 1972). A short fermentation like Run 36 (Table 8.1) can collapse, but this must not happen in a fermentation intended to run for 12 or more days.

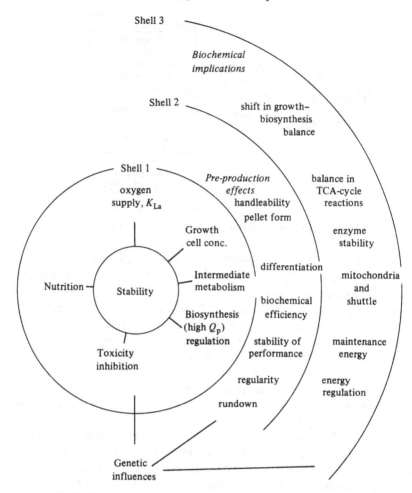

Fig. 10.5. Aspects of maximum antibiotic production.

Shell 2 lists some of the factors vital to successful preparation of the inoculum, on which success depends. The stylised diagram in Fig. 3.9d shows an initial charge of 5 g of cells/l which implies a highly developed and concentrated inoculum culture. Some of the aspects listed here are discussed in Part 1. The form of pellets produced and their biochemical activity are of particular importance. This subject is reviewed by Demain & Solomon (1986, pp. 32–40).

The outer shell (3) lists a few points likely to be important biochemically. These include adaptation to the new pattern of metabolism suggested in Fig. 10.4. The balance in the TCA cycle reactions must be important, since much energy is being diverted to antibiotic synthesis. Synthesis of amino acids via the TCA cycle must also be important, with catabolism also occurring. In fungi, the situation is different, as these processes are separated in the mitochondria and cytoplasm and will involve different types of regulation. If the TCA cycle goes out of balance, intermediates like succinate could accumulate, with serious effects on the overall system.

Fig. 10.5 also draws attention to the fact that genetic regulation is involved in all the shells. The microorganisms likely to be in use at this stage of development may have been greatly changed from the natural state, and this could interfere with attempts to rationalise the fermentation process.

The suggestions made in Fig. 10.5 are only a few of those that might occur to an expert considering a situation of this sort, but they give an idea of some of the features important to the situation.

Summarising the position, it is seen that to move to a new situation, it is necessary (1) to gain an idea of how the new fermentations would behave, and what their requirements would be, especially the requirement for oxygen, (2) to discover how to produce a stable cell population that is capable of long-term operation without growth, and in a form that would not restrict oxygen transfer, and (3) to devise feed and control programmes that would ensure a stable operating sytem. In the succeeding sections an attempt will be made to indicate literature examples that indicate how these requirements can be met.

10.5.2   Limits to production

The introduction has already brought out factors important to success. Many of these are summarised in Fig. 10.5. These are expressed in general terms. In development work it would be necessary at the start to work out particular factors that were already limiting the fermentation under study, and that would have to be removed before progress could be made. These might involve aspects of the strain that made progress difficult, for example poor sporulation, which would have to be overcome by special sub-culture routines, or sensitivity to the antibiotic or other products, which would have to be overcome. Priority would have to be given to these matters before other work could be done.

10.5.3   Oxygen requirements and the effect of enzyme decay

Oxygen transfer is a critical factor in fermentations that are aimed at maximal levels of production, and the fermentation has to be adjusted to work within this limitation. This is particularly so with penicillin, because antibiotic synthesis itself requires such large amounts of energy. It is therefore necessary to understand its effect on the situation, and to assess the implications of enzyme decay.

Since data from batches giving maximum yields are not available, it is necessary to approach the subject using a model. The model given in

Table 8.3 is suitable for this purpose, with certain modifications. As large and differing amounts of penicillin are to be considered, the term p was calculated from the known requirement for oxygen for synthesis. Requirements per gram were assumed to be 0.4 l for cells (i.e. $Y = 2.5$), and 2.2 l for penicillin, based on the literature data. The maintenance constant (m) was set at 0.006. Instead of developing a growth curve by means of an equation, a value for dx/dt was inserted for each 10-h step, so that any shape could be produced. Although penicillin was calculated in units(u), it was converted to g/l, for convenience, using the relationship 1 mg penicillin $= 1666$ u. In considering the results obtained from the model, it will be appreciated that it is only an approximation to reality and depends on assumptions that are subject to error.

The results of the investigations are given in Table 10.7. Three growth patterns are used. The first is like that in Run 30 (Fig. 3.3a). The second is similar to that given by Queener & Swartz (1979) in their Fig. 5, with rapid growth on the first day, then a slower pattern. The third follows the stylised pattern of Fig. 3.9d, the growth curve up to 50 h being synthesised using the logistic law equation (Fig. 8.1), with an initial cell concentration of 5 g/l.

Each type of batch was tested using different production rates (Q_p) and decay constants (E). The effect of different values of E are given at the foot of Table 10.7.

The results in the first row of the Run 30 series shows a general similarity to Run 30 itself, thus confirming the model. To obtain high production it was necessary to increase Q_p and reduce E. With the second set, the second row agrees with the original batch illustrated by Queener & Swartz (1979), and the other rows show batches with different conditions. With the stylised fermentations, titres were maximal, mainly due to the very low decay coefficient used, which gave an almost linear production curve.

A low decay coefficient was one of the most important factors in obtaining high yields during prolonged fermentations. The high decay factor in Run 30 makes prolonged production impossible and therefore limits the possibility of maximisation. Provided the decay constant is low, a value of Q_p of 15 or 20 can give very good results, i.e. 2–3 times the levels obtained 25 years ago. The advances have partly been in Q_p, but importantly, they have also been in increased resistance to decay. This decay may be due to loss of the enzymes, but it is also likely to be due to increased resistance to product inhibition.

The production of maximum yields is associated with high demands for oxygen. These increase from about 0.55 l/l/h with the Run 30 fermentation, to 1.0–1.5 l/l/h with maximum yields. This may be an over-estimate, as the current best strains are probably more efficient than those on which the model was based. The Queener & Swartz examples

Table 10.7. Oxygen requirements for penicillin production, high and maximum yields

Type of batch	Growth pattern Age (h)	Cell conc. (g/l)	Q_P (u/g/h)	Decay constant (E)	Penicillin (g/l) 120 h	180 h	240 h	Oxygen uptake (l/l/h) 40 h	80 h	150 h	240 h
(1) 'Run 30'	20	11	7.5	0.015	6.5	—	—	0.56	0.52	—	—
	30	22	7.5	0.005	12.9	19.1	23.7	0.63	0.69	0.54	0.45
	50	35	15	0.005	25.7	38.2	47.4	0.87	1.00	0.78	0.60
	100+	50	20	0.005	34.5	50.9	63.2	1.02	1.21	0.94	0.70
(2) Queener & Swartz	20	20	10	0.015	7.4(100 h)			0.49	0.41	—	—
	30	25	12	0.015	10.0	11.1(150 h)		0.53	0.44	0.32	—
	50	31	12	0.005	18.9	23.3(150 h)		0.66	0.66	0.56	—
	100+	42	20	0.005	31.6	45.2	55.3	0.92	0.93	0.77	0.58
(3) 'Stylised'	20	18	12	0.0015	32.3	50.0	66.1	1.16	1.05	0.975	0.89
	30	30	20	0.015	21.4	—	—	1.14	0.70	—	—
	50	48	20	0.005	41	57.5	69.5	1.43	1.19	0.93	0.70
	100+	50	25	0.0015	66.3	102.0	—	1.83	1.80	1.65	—
(4) Oxytetracycline			Q_{OTC}		Oxytetracycline (g/l)						
Growth: slowed stylised, 45 g/l at 60 h, 50 g/l at 80 h			7	0.0015	23.6	40.3	55.5	.71	.36	.34	.32

$m = 0.003$, $K = 0.77$,
$p = p/2$, $E = 0.0015$,
$Q = 7$,
1 mg OTC = 1000u
Growth: slowed stylised, 45 g/l
at 60 h, 50 g/l at 80 h

Parameters: oxygen, 0.4 l/g cells; 2.2 l/g penicillin; $m = 0.006$; 1 mg penicillin = 1666 units.
Decay effect at 150 h ($e^{-T.E}$): $E = 0.015$, 0.11; $E = 0.005$, 0.47; $E = 0.0015$, 0.80.

seem more economical, but the cell concentration was lower. Taking a value of 1.2 l/l/h, and a minimum concentration of dissolved oxygen of 33% saturation, this would require a value of 324/h for the transfer coefficient K_{La}, with a cell concentration of 50 g/l. Well-stirred laboratory fermenters, in general, would only reach half this figure at this cell concentration. It is evident that prolonged fermentations are needed for maximum results, to spread out the requirement for oxygen so as to meet availability.

A single oxytetracycline batch is shown in Table 10.7, using the parameters given in Table 3.2 to calculate oxygen requirements. For the production stage, oxygen demands were low, but it was necessary to slow down early growth so as to avoid excessive oxygen demands. This was allowed for in the example given.

10.5.4   Increase of production by modification of the fermentation system
Introduction
The previous sections have shown that the move to maximal production requires changes in the design of the fermentation system, so as to provide higher specific productivity, resistance of the biosynthetic enzymes to decay and repression, and growth in a form that will allow the required amount of oxygen to reach the mycelium. Also needed are fermentations in which growth metabolism is stabilised and restricted, so that the main material flow is directed to antibiotic biosynthesis. It is not possible to define the precise way in which this can be done, but examples are available to illustrate possible routes to the desired objectives.

Oxygen transfer in different cultures
Three penicillin batches, two of which have already been described, provide data for a consideration of this subject (Calam & Ismail, 1980). The results are shown in Table 10.8. The three batches show significantly different behaviour with respect to oxygen transfer (K_{La}). The synthetic medium seems most promising, with peanut medium somewhat better than corn-steep medium. Experience also suggests that the production enzymes were more stable in the batch with synthetic medium. This suggests the possibility of developing a process of the desired type, though a synthetic medium would probably not be the ultimate solution.

Increases in production by modification of growth
It is convenient to deal with this question by quoting a number of examples in which the desired characteristics have been induced successfully, at least at the experimental level.

Citric acid: Citric acid has long been manufactured on a very large scale by a fermentation process using *Aspergillus niger* to ferment sucrose or

Table 10.8. *Parameters from three laboratory batches*

Run	Medium	Age: (h)	40	60	80	100	120	Average CO_2 output rates (l/l/h)
30	corn steep	Cells (g/l)	32	39	43	46	47	0.48
		K_{La} (h^{-1})	140	167	175	138	114	
		DOT (% sat.)	37	55	50	40	25	
9	synthetic	Cells (g/l)	30	40	55	40[a]	55	1.13
		K_{La} (h^{-1})	430	480	315	650	470	
		DOT (% sat.)	65	50	35	70	55	
36	peanut meal	Cells (g/l) (insol.)	48	50	57	66	76	0.84
		Cells (g/l) (calc.)	25	38	52	59	65	
		K_{La} (h^{-1})	170	330	205	226	197	
		DOT (% sat.)	45	42	28	33	20	

[a] Diluted.

cane juice to the acid. The process was originally operated in surface culture, but in the 1940s a submerged fermentation process was developed. The fermentation is interesting in that 75–80% conversions can be obtained industrially, under favourable conditions. This involves the forcing of primary metabolism to overproduce an intermediate substance, citric acid, and it is this aspect that is important here, since this action is needed to increase antibiotic production. In early experiments, Shu & Johnson (1945) obtained high yields in shaken flasks. It was noted that the concentration of phosphate was an important factor in obtaining the best results. Later workers (e.g. Miles Laboratories Inc., 1952) described the optimal form of pellets that was important for high yields. These were small and consisted of radiating, thickened hyphae. At the time there was considerable controversy about the best form of pellets and the best conditions, but it is now evident that individual strains require individual optimal conditions. The best results are obtained when the fungus grows in an optimal mycelial form, with growth restricted by the phosphate concentration, and with certain inorganic ions (such as Fe, Mn, and others) at carefully adjusted levels. This limits TCA cycle activity while allowing extensive production of citrate, using oxalacetate from a supplementary pathway as precursor, as illustrated in Fig. 4.1. It is interesting that the control of growth by phosphate limitation is used to maximise antibiotic fermentations (Chapter 3.6). There is an extensive literature on citric acid production, both by *A. niger* and by certain yeasts.

Although the citric acid fermentation does not resemble an antibiotic fermentation, it is instructive as it shows the enzyme system locked into a particular form that causes the cells to produce a particular substance in large amounts, and that resembles an immobilised form of the enzyme mechanism.

Penicillin – König et al. *(1982)*: In a series of experiments, the possibility of penicillin production was investigated using an aerated tower fermenter with re-cycle to improve aeration and mixing. An industrial strain was used, Hoechst H 617/S1, and the production medium contained lactose, sucrose, cotton-seed flour (Pharmamedia), calcium carbonate, sodium thiosulphate, and phenoxyacetic acid. A proprietary antifoam agent was used.

The inoculum was grown in a glucose + lactose + corn-steep medium, with calcium carbonate and ammonium sulphate, in a 50-l fermenter, stirred at 520 rpm by turbine agitators. Cell concentrations were measured by passing the samples through a fine sieve, which enabled separation of cells from chalk and residual Pharmamedia.

Working in the manner described, the culture produced a thick mass of sludge. Dissolved oxygen fell to 3% of saturation by 50 h, and penicillin reached only 0.5 g/l by 150 h.

It was found that if the stirring speed in the inoculum fermenter was reduced to 200 rpm, small pellets were formed. In the fermenter, growth continued to be in the form of small pellets, and the cell concentration reached 30 g/l, remaining constant up to 150 h with dissolved oxygen at 30–40% of saturation, and with penicillin reaching the expected level of 3.5 g/l.

Further tests with the inoculum fermenter showed the following results:

rpm	Form of growth
200	large pellets, 0.6–2 mm diameter, hollow
400	small pellets, below 0.6 mm diameter
600	filaments

The small pellets obtained at 400 rpm grew quite well in the fermenter, but it was necessary to reduce the strength of the medium. This gave a cell concentration of 20 g/l and sub-optimal penicillin production. Pellets grown at 200 rpm proved more stable than the others, giving a low viscosity culture, which would be expected to save expense industrially as regards the cost of stirring and cooling.

Penicillin – Hockenhull & McKenzie (1986): The original fed-batch process for penicillin production was referred to earlier (Hosler & Johnson, 1952). It is based on a synthetic medium, with glucose feed and pH control with ammonia. Industrial experience showed that this was not always reliable, and it was preferred to use corn-steep liquor as a basis, together with a feed of sugar. It was possible to adjust this feed so as to provide just enough sugar to maintain the cells in good condition and to produce penicillin. Too little sugar diminished biosynthesis, while too much caused excessive growth.

With the synthetic medium system, the main problem was the transition from the early growth phase to the later condition with production and little growth. If this was mishandled, production was low and continued for only a short time. By studying the growth pattern obtained with corn-steep medium, the ideal sugar-feed pattern to copy it was derived. A good copy could be obtained using the logistic law model, with a doubling time of 5.5 h. An illustrative batch is presented, using a very-high-yielding industrial strain and a basic medium containing calcium carbonate, potassium phosphate, ammonium sulphate, mineral salts, and vegetable oil, together with a planned feed of sugar. The batch gave results equal to one with corn-steep liquor, with the cell concentration, after an initial growth period from 0–40 h, almost constant till 180 h. There was a constant rate of penicillin production from 20–180 h.

One of the most interesting features of this batch was the long-term, continuous production of penicillin while the cell concentration remained constant. A method of culture that provided stable production conditions while allowing a high level of oxygen transfer had evidently been found. This foreshadowed the maximum yield system, illustrated in Fig. 3.9d.

Novobiocin – Ross & Wilkin (1966): The production of novobiocin, using *Streptomyces griseus* in a continuous flow tower fermenter, was described. The medium contained corn-steep liquor and glucose. During the first 7 days of cultivation, before the flow was started, the streptomycete grew in a filamentous form, but soon after the feed was started, the culture changed to a particulate, granular condition. This allowed good aeration and production of novobiocin. The first claim in the patent was a method of culture giving a particulate and aeratable form. In the example, there was very slow growth during the continuous culture, from 27 g/l at day 10 to 35 g/l at day 27, with novobiocin steady at approximately 520 mg/l in the outflow.

Other fermentations with special features: The following fermentations have already been described in Section 10.4.2: cephalosporin C, where a special growth-form is important for high production; and griseofulvin and gibberellic acid, where carefully controlled feeds are employed to keep production going for periods up to 300–400 h.

Pellet formation in antibiotic fermentations: This is a subject that has been much discussed in the literature, and there is no space here for a review. Changes in penicillin-production culture have been described by Duckworth & Harris (1949) and by Righelato *et al.* (1968). In these and other papers, mycelial behaviour was correlated with productivity, growth, and morphology. Much other work (for example by Professor N. W. F. Kossen and collaborators at Delft) has been directed to an understanding of the relation between morphology, viscosity, and oxygen transfer, from a biochemical engineering standpoint.

Discussion
The object here has been to present information on the way in which the characteristics of a fermentation can be assessed and directed to a situation when maximum production becomes possible.

The information provided by the calculations and the examples indicates approaches that have led to the type of maximised fermentations (summarised in the graphs in Fig. 3.9d) that give stable production with minimum growth, and adequate transfer of oxygen. This implies the selection of mutants that are capable of growing in the correct form and resisting product inhibition, and then the designing of the appropriate culture conditions to optimise their use. To carry out a programme of this type would involve every aspect of microbiology, as described in previous chapters, and would require well-planned and detailed research over a long period. The dating of the references given above show that the current maximal results have arisen from a long period of expert development, beginning in the era of high yields and leading through various further stages of productivity.

The transfer of processes of this type to the main plant would raise a number of problems. The highly stirred and aerated conditions in the plant might affect the formation and behaviour of the type of pellets preferred, and it might take some time and effort before the necessary ideal growth and production conditions could be discovered.

10.6　General approach to development

As will be seen from this account, process improvement starts empirically and then moves towards a more and more systematic approach, based on a detailed understanding of the factors involved. Each problem is different, but it is possible to make a generalised approach to the subjects.

In the present case, the analysis of the problem has been based on a limited number of ideas. Other workers might be inclined to stress other concepts, especially the application of genetics. This widening is to be greatly encouraged. The researcher should therefore study the literature and examine the views of experts. It will be realised that academic workers usually express their ideas in detail, but with industrial workers the key statement is often tucked away in a remote paragraph, or even omitted.

In the analysis of a problem, it is often helpful to express the complex of ideas in some sort of model, not necessarily mathematical. This enables new ideas to be tested, and it enables areas of agreement and disagreement between model and experimental conclusions to be identified, thus enabling a better understanding of the problem. The importance of identifying and quantifying limits is very great. Product inhibition has been stressed, but this is not always the primary limiter, and it would be wasteful to attack the wrong limiter. This problem can only be tackled by a careful study of the fermentation, often by the development of special experimental techniques. In the end, it is the design of a critical experiment that provides the step forward.

It may become important to select and develop new strains that will have the properties that will be needed to make maximisation a possibility. Such a programme would inevitably take a long time, and this would have serious management implications.

The need for maximisation arises from a number of directions, mainly to cheapen prices and to increase supplies. Although the possibility of purchasing material exists and is often practiced, pharmaceutical firms usually prefer to be able to offer their own products for sale, while dependence on purchase can involve difficulties over quality and availability. At the moment, British firms seem to be tending to increase capacity by building new plants or extending old ones.

Certain aspects of development are brought out by the following two lines, listing the main process stages:

(a) Strain; pre-production stages (inoculum); production stage.

(b) Production stages; pre-production stages (inoculum); strain.

During progress to high yields, the first listing expresses the main line of thought, i.e. a good strain has been obtained, and the later stages must be optimised to take advantage of it. Later, in maximisation, the limits of the production stage become fixed by oxygen transfer limits and biochemical requirements. The object is how to make the best use of the production stage, and the strain and the pre-production stages must be optimised to achieve this purpose. At any point it might be worth writing, on separate sheets of paper, the words: strain: pre-production stages: production stage, and then adding to each the details that need settlement for optimal results. There may be little to write at first, but later some highly complex ideas may appear on each of the pages.

It may be concluded that process development will remain necessary. Management would probably prefer to let this be done in house, but there are other options. These include the purchase of new strains from firms like Pan Labs or CETUS. Alternatively, these firms will develop one of the firm's strains, taking advantage of their equipment and expertise. Purchase or contract development may prove very expensive, but it could be argued to be well worth the money. Although this may seem unattractive to the local team, it has to be considered as a possibly rapid road to success.

Part 3

Industrial fermentation plants and pilot plants

The move from development in the laboratory or research pilot plant to development in the main plant involves very considerable changes in methods and ideas. These arise mainly from the size of the equipment, but also from the very different approach that is necessary in commercial operations. In a way, it can be said that the laboratory worker is usually free to think and to experiment and to regard the fermentation process as flexible. Some experiments work and are followed up, others do not do so well and are forgotten. As the work moves to the main plant, the assumption is that the process is now clearly defined, and the objective is to bring it into operation with a minimum of risk, without embarking on a series of experiments. In any case, in large-scale work, the idea of discarding a batch is unthinkable on account of the expense. Thus the introduction of a new process to the plant requires a programme that is well thought out and very reliable, and fully backed up by laboratory work.

In this connection, the main role of the pilot plant is to check laboratory processes as well as possible to establish their suitability for plant work. The larger pilot-plant fermenters may be used for this (1000–5000 l), as well as for producing kilogram quantities of new substances for test.

The role of the main plant is commercial, i.e. to produce quantities of material for sale at a profit. The firm's profitability, and the availability of cash resources for research and development, depend upon the success of the main plant. Plant management appreciates the value of research, but the plant is not built for research, nor does it provide facilities for it. Its staff structure is commercial and much of the staff's time is devoted to works administration and operation. The introduction of process improvements has to fit into this situation, and a process development programme has to be adapted to these conditions.

Because of the way commercial pilot plants and main plants operate, the wealth of information available in a research laboratory, from highly instrumented fermenters, will probably not be available. At the same time, the methods used in plant work and the nature of large-scale fermentations can introduce new problems in development work. These

149

can include difficulties in reproducibility due to difficulties of standardising inocula and the variations produced by constant changes in the medium ingredients used, week by week. Therefore, the discussion of process development at plant level has to take into account these problems.

It is clearly not possible here to give a detailed account of the design and operation of large fermentation plants. All that is attempted is to give a broad description of a fermentation plant, its working, and the activities of the various departments involved in plant operations. It is an attempt to indicate to young researchers who are becoming involved in plant development what plants are like, how they are operated, and how to approach research into their problems, if they happen to arise.

Although the circumstances are different when development research is conducted in the laboratory and in the plant, especially in space and time and in the way the work is organised, it should be stressed that scientifically the approaches and the considerations are the same.

11 Fermentation plants and pilot plants

11.1 The antibiotics factory

Although antibiotics process development is concerned with the fermentation stage of manufacture, it forms part of the activities of a group of works units which involve all stages of production. It is therefore important to appreciate the scope of the activities that are included in a typical antibiotics factory. It is likely that such a plant will include the following facilities or work areas.
  (a) Basic physical inputs: steam raising, electricity, water, and effluent disposal.
  (b) Laboratories for analysis and for the production of seed cultures for the fermentation plant.
  (c) The fermentation building and its ancillary equipment.
  (d) Development facilities, often in the form of a pilot plant.
  (e) Filtration and extraction buildings.
  (f) Plant for the preparation of pharmaceutical products for sale.
  (g) Engineering maintenance facilities of various types.
  (h) Management and administration.
Works buildings are commonly referred to as 'sheds'. This has no derogatory significance, and will be adopted in later descriptions.
  All these facilities are of great importance for success, and have their own operational methods and considerations. For example, steam, electricity, and water are used to a very large extent, each costing millions of pounds per year. Water is important for cooling the fermenters, and it is often necessary to provide for the cooling of the water and for re-cycling, especially in warm weather, to make effective use of it. One plant employs a large refrigeration system for this purpose. Many plants have to provide treatment units to bring down the biological oxygen requirement of the effluent before it can be discharged. The purification of the products and the pharmaceutical and sales side must also be stressed, as they involve a great deal of detailed work. Typically, the bulk of the products are exported, and the assembly and despatch of the consignments requires a major planning effort. Mechanically, the plant includes thousands of valves, instruments, and control systems, and a great deal of effort is needed to keep them all in order.
  Fig. 11.1, kindly provided by Beecham Pharmaceuticals, UK Division (Worthing, Sussex), illustrates such a fermentation plant that carries out all manufacturing stages. These include steam generation, fermentation

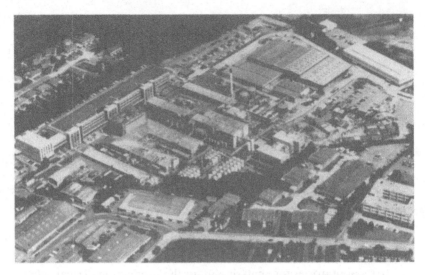

Fig. 11.1. Beecham Pharmaceutical's antibiotics factory, Worthing, Sussex.

broth production, filtration, and extraction. Extraction requires a tank farm for solvent dispersion and recovery, this being important economically. Other buildings contain the pharmaceutical and packaging plant, stores, warehouses, engineering maintenance, and other support activities. It will be realised that such a plant requires stocks of all kinds of materials, implying an extensive support organisation.

One of the main points brought out by Fig. 11.1 is the scale and complexity of the plant, all parts of which involve high technologies. The successful operation of the plant obviously requires very good administration and management. It will also be seen that fermentation is only one of many important activities in the works. Although fermentation process development appears to relate only to the fermentation plant, experience shows that it soon becomes involved with the operations of the rest of the works, and this can greatly increase the interest of this field of activity.

11.2   A visit to a fermentation plant

The main points likely to be seen during a visit will be described briefly to indicate the nature of the operations involved in the production of the crude, extracted antibiotic. On visits, it is evident that freedom from infection is always a main objective; visitors wear sterile clothing and sometimes are only shown the plant from enclosed viewing stations.

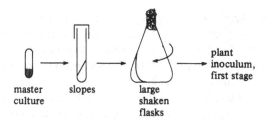

Fig. 11.2. Preparation of seed for plant batches.

11.2.1   The seed culture

The first visit is usually to the seed preparation unit, where the starting cultures for the plant process are prepared. A high level of sterility is always to be seen. The stages involved are shown in Fig. 11.2. These operations are conducted in a large and specially planned work area. Key areas are supplied with sterile air, and all entrants wear sterile clothing and shoes.

The outer areas are usually 'dirty'; this is where used apparatus is sterilised, washed, and prepared for use with the necessary media. All the equipment is then placed in a double-ended steriliser. After sterilisation, the equipment is unloaded into the sterile area. At one end of the sterile area there is usually a bench supplied with laminar-flow, sterile air; this is where the main operations are conducted.

The master culture is usually held freeze-dried, or in liquid nitrogen. The tubes are used to inoculate slopes, and these, in turn, are used to start large shaken-flask cultures, for example 1–2 l of medium in 5-l flasks. The optimal method of working, at this stage, will have been determined experimentally. The seed culture, which grows after a few days, may be in the form of pellets or spores, depending on the organism used. The seed flasks are incubated on a high-speed shaker located within the sterile area. The flasks are usually closed by special aseptic closures.

When ready, the flasks are returned to the working area and the culture is transferred to a steel transfer bottle. This consists of a stainless-steel vessel, 5–10 l in capacity, fitted with an outlet pipe and coupling for attachment to a sterilised coupling on the inoculum fermenter. The culture or cultures are poured aseptically into the transfer vessel, which is then ready for use. The seed may be held for a limited time in the refrigerator.

11.2.2   The inoculum or pre-production stage

As the visit proceeds, the visitors now move up to the fermentation area, which requires an ascent of several floors by lift. The inocula are grown in

a special area, which is kept as clean as possible. The upper parts of 500-l
and 5000-l fermenters may be seen; these are for the first and second (or
more) stages of growth. The fermenters are similar to production
fermenters. The first step may take 30–48 h; the second stage may take
less. The final inoculum culture is checked as to its readiness for transfer
to the production fermenter. In a large plant with 20–30 main fermenters,
inoculations and harvestings take place several times per day, so there is
a considerable amount of work to be done.

The transfer of inocula is carried out using a special system of pipelines.
These are usually held filled with steam under pressure. This is referred to
as a steam lock. Great care has to be taken over the design of these
pipelines, so as to avoid the accumulation of culture or water in the lines,
or the occurrence of pockets, which may be very difficult to sterilise. The
successful preparation of inocula requires considerable skill and attention
to detail. Although the system may seem straightforward, with
operations performed in a calm manner, it is a critical step for high yields,
as regards both freedom from infection and productivity.

11.2.3   The fermentation shed

To go from the inoculum area to the fermenter hall involves a
considerable change. This is often because of the great increase in noise.
While some plants are quiet, others may require the use of ear-muffs. The
noise is usually due to the gearboxes in the stirrer drive system. The
airflow and stirrer system involves several thousand horsepower in a plant
with about 20 fermenters of 100-m^3 capacity, each with several hundred
horsepower, and this causes vibration and a feeling of swaying. This
produces an other-worldly atmosphere, often increased by the absence of
any other human beings, except the visitors.

The domed tops of the fermenters are usually raised somewhat above
floor level. There is a central tower supporting the drive. A number of
pipes, large and small and each with control valves, enter the top of the
fermenter. These supply air, cooling water, and steam, along with feeds,
additions, antifoam, and pH control. The air and cooling systems are
extensive, and the necessary pipework may be visible or may be partly
concealed in supply channels. The large size of the control valves will be
noticed, emphasising the problem of sterilising them. Another set of
installations is the air filters. These are often quite large, cylindrical
bodies, filled with glass fibre, but there is a tendency to use cartridge-type
filters, containing a ceramic element, which are smaller. The reason why
the visitor finds himself on the fourth floor is because of the tallness of the
fermenters. Other equipment may be located on lower floors.

In former times, the instrumentation was a prominent feature. This is
nowadays more and more centralised, but there are often small panels
near each fermenter, giving the key information. The system allows

manual control in the event of the failure of the main computer. These small panels may also be seen in the inoculum area. A large panel may also be seen, showing the status of each fermenter, and showing alarm lights if attention is needed.

A visit to a fermentation shed is interesting to the visitor mainly in giving an idea of the scale and complexity of the fermentation unit, and the degree of engineering design and development that must have gone into it. It will also show the high level of organisation required to keep such a production system in good operating condition. The extent to which a development researcher should know about the details of a plant and its operation is arguable, but it is useful to have a good idea of the nature of a plant, and to spend time in studying its details and the way it is run, and to discover its possibilities and limitations. It is also useful to learn how its operators see it and how they express their views about how it should be run. Without this information, it may be difficult, in discussion, to understand what is meant and to appreciate what a change in working methods would mean in practice.

11.2.4   The control room

The management is sometimes rather unwilling to allow access to visitors to the control room, for fear of exposing too much detail about operational details and ideas.

Originally, each fermenter had its own instruments and recorders (temperature, airflow, etc.), and feed arrangements were also worked manually. Records of the pH and other details were written hourly on special sheets. This recording system involved considerable labour, for example in changing recorder charts and circulating them. The abstraction of batch details later often proved difficult and time consuming. In the course of time, following the examples of the chemical and petroleum industries, this instrumentation was moved to a central control room. Many of the manually operated valves were replaced by servo-operated types, worked also from the control room, where recording was centralised. These ideas were expanded when computers came into use, facilitating these procedures.

At the present time, comprehensive computer control systems are used, similar to those described in Chapter 7.7 on laboratory work. Provided with the details, these systems will set and prepare the fermenter and operate all the necessary controls and additions, such as feeds and antifoam. In the event of a malfunction, an alarm will be given, and the supervisor can turn to the computer to identify and correct the fault. The computer also stores and lists data. There have been many developments in control methods over the last 20 years (Society of Chemical Industry, 1986), and current ideas are discussed below (Section 11.3.6).

The use of computer systems of this kind have had a considerable effect on fermenter operation. In former times each shift involved a group of trained process men under the control of a foreman who directed the work programme. The foreman also noted the data coming from the fermenter instruments and made such changes as seemed necessary. Advice might be sought from analysts or the manager, if available. At present, the process men tend to plan their own work schedules as a group, while the foreman, after training, has become a supervisor who operates the plant on the basis of the computer system.

Although centralised control rooms are generally provided, the degree of automatic control that is used varies, and in some plants, control is mainly manual. This point will be discussed later.

11.2.5   Medium make-up

On returning to ground level, a visit may be made to the area where media are made. The details of this process vary greatly; some procedures are automated, while others work in a much simpler way.

The process begins with an ingredients list for the batch being prepared, and the materials are obtained from an adjacent warehouse. After being weighed they are loaded on pallets in bags and then taken for loading into the fermenter, or to a mixing vessel for solution before being transferred to the fermenter for making up to volume. In one, more-elaborate case, the ingredients list appeared on an illuminated panel, and the process man assigned each weighed amount to a mixing vessel, in the correct order. The mixing tank was mounted on a load cell that checked the weight of each addition. If correct, the item disappeared from the panel, notifying readiness for the next addition. The additions might involve automatic weighing and delivery from a silo, or the separate additions of smaller portions.

11.2.6   Filtration and extraction

On completion of a batch and approval for extraction, the fermenter contents are usually passed to a cooled holding vessel of similar size, so that the preparation of the next batch can begin without delay. In some cases anaerobic fermentation can occur, leading to heating in the storage vessel and hence the need for cooling.

The culture is then passed to the filter, often via a small mixing tank where addition of filter aid and coagulant chemicals may be made to facilitate filtration. In some cases, pH adjustment may be necessary to bring the product into solution; in a few cases, the separated mycelium is kept and extracted. Also, in some cases, the whole culture is passed up a column of ion-exchange resin particles to recover the product, as with streptomycin. Filtration is usually by means of a rotary vacuum filter. This consists of a perforated drum covered with a special cloth. The cloth may be used alone, or covered with a thick layer of diatomaceous filter aid. The drum, which slowly rotates, dips into a large trough, to which the culture is fed. Reduced pressure sucks the culture fluid into the drum, through the filter cloth, and it is subsequently pumped out for extraction. If the cloth is used alone, it passes over an extra roller that causes the mycelium to drop off into a skip. If filter aid is used, the rotating drum passes a knife that scrapes off the mycelium and some of the filter aid; this provides a new surface for filtration.

The antibiotic is recovered from the filtration with solvents such as butyl acetate or butanol. As a rule, special centrifugal counterflow machines are used to give good separation of culture broth and solvent. The product is then isolated chemically in a nearly pure form. It may be dried in a vacuum oven or by hot air, depending on its stability, and it is then stored in drums for further purification as a pharmaceutical preparation.

The ease and efficiency of the filtration and recovery process depends on the quality of the fermentation process, and this is a factor that has to be taken into account in fermentation development work. It has to be realised that the filtration, extraction, and purification processes also involves high levels of technology.

11.3   The main plant units involved in commercial fermentations

As will be seen, a fermentation plant is a complex organisation. The nucleus is provided by the fermenters, but these are supplemented by many other systems, such as the sterile-air system, culture-transfer pipes, steam and electricity supplies, and the cooling-water system. Each of these implies engineering maintenance groups. Along with these go medium preparation, sterilisation, the control system, and many others. Of these systems, fermentation development research is involved mainly with the fermenters, the sterile-air supply, and the pipework used to supply the inoculum and feed additions, i.e. the sterile materials transfer systems. The others are important practically and economically, but mainly indirectly. The fermenters, sterile-air system, and the transfer pipework will therefore be discussed here. The cooling-water system is also important, and often critical, as in some places the water may be too warm and insufficient, thus causing problems in temperature control. Some water supplies may also be corrosive. While the researcher may have to recognise this problem, it is not a factor that he is likely to be able to do anything about. A fourth subject that will also be discussed is the sterilisation of the plant. It will only be possible to touch on the more-obvious aspects of these subjects; those requiring more detail must look elsewhere.

There is another aspect of works operations that must be kept in mind.

Table 11.1. *Main stages in an antibiotic production batch*

Stage	Working staff	Time (days)
Preparation of working slopes from master culture	microbiology	10
5-l shaken-flask seed	laboratory	
cultures		2–3
First inoculum stage, stirred fermenter, 0.5 m³		1.5–2
Second inoculum stage, stirred fermenter, 5 m³	plant staff	0.5–1
Main production stage, stirred fermenter, 100 m³		5–15
		Total 27 approx.

An extra stage, taking several days, might be needed between the working slope and the seed flasks.

Works operate according to daily, weekly, or monthly plans, so that tests and alterations to fermenter conditions may, with the best will in the world, take some time to organise.

The cost of a fermenter, in terms of the total installation, has been given as £27/l by Rowlands & Normansell (1983).

11.3.1   Outline of plant process
The main steps involved in the conduct of a plant batch, and the time required, are shown in Table 11.1.

11.3.2   Industrial fermenters
Description
A fermentation shed may contain 20 or more large fermenters. The working capacity of these fermenters is usually quoted as 100 m³, and this will be assumed here. Sizes vary in different places, and 120-m³ fermenters have been seen in some installations. The shape of the fermenters is relatively standard, the height : diameter ratio being 3 : 1. In operation, part of this is left free to provide head space, the height : diameter ratio for the culture being 2.5 : 1. Assuming 100 m³ of culture this gives a diameter of 3.7 m and a total height of 11.1 m, to which must be added 2–3 m for the drive plus a working space above the fermenter. This explains why fermentation sheds are so high. Fermenters are usually made of stainless steel, but mild steel has often been used for this purpose.

It is difficult to give an impression of a fermenter, but the tall, aluminium-covered tanks often seen around brewery buildings give an impression of the shape and size.

When the fermenter is working, the culture is filled with air bubbles, causing expansion, and there may be a metre of foam. For this reason, ample head space is needed.

On looking into the interior of a fermenter, through the manhole, cooling coils are seen near the walls, and the walls themselves may have half-circular coils welded on the outside to increase the cooling area. The stirrers have a diameter one third to one half the vessel diameter, and they consist of a disc fitted with blades on the outer edge, or curved turbine blades fixed to a boss. In a large fermenter, three stirrers are fitted on the shaft, one above the other. This provides three zones of vigorous agitation, separated from each other. Although this would be expected to give poor overall vertical mixing, results are satisfactory. Air is admitted to the bottom of the fermenter via one to two open pipes, sometimes by special jets. Steam for sterilisation is admitted by the air pipes. Baffles are attached to the sides of the fermenter and are about one twentieth of its diameter. The stirrer shaft enters the fermenter through a mechanical seal held by steam pressure, and it is steadied by bearings in the fermenter.

A number of pipes enter the fermenter, providing the air supply, cooling water, and various feeds. There is also a sampling point and connections to add inoculum to the fermenter. Also noticeable will be the cables attached to the various probes and instruments that are used for the control of the system.

During a short visit, it is not difficult to get a general appreciation of the system. If research is involved, it is usually necessary to go further and obtain a good understanding of the layout, and the way it is controlled and operated. This requires time for observation and reflection.

Efficiency of stirring and agitation, and culture limitations
The design of industrial fermenters is usually put into the hands of specialist firms who have a knowledge of the requirements of most types of fermentations. These requirements are usually similar to those for laboratory work, i.e. good mixing and an adequate oxygen transfer rate. A minimal value for this, 4 g/l/h, by the sulphite method, has been mentioned previously (Chapter 3.3.7), and this can usually be achieved by a standard fermenter, provided the power input is sufficient. Early workers Wegrich & Schurter (1953), who investigated the penicillin fermentation in fermenters with capacities of 2000 and 24 000 US gallons, considered 0.7 horsepower (hp)/100 US gallons to be optimal. More recently, Queener & Swartz (1979) considered 0.61 hp/100 US gallons to be too low for this fermentation. This lower value might be sufficient for oxytetracycline production (cf. Chapter 3.5) as this fermentation requires considerably less oxygen. At 1 hp/100 US gallons, a 100-m^3 fermenter would hold 28 000 US gallons (22 500 imperial gallons) and require 280 hp, or approximately 250 kW, providing some extra power to allow for losses in the gears etc. The adequacy of stirring can therefore be

estimated by looking at the specification plate on the motor, but it would be necessary to establish whether the motor was being used at full power or not. At a given rate of stirring, the power requirement is influenced by the airflow rate, nearly doubling in the absence of air. To allow for this, two-speed gearboxes are used so as to allow slow stirring during sterilisation, and in some cases variable speed drives are used.

In plant work the airflow rate is usually about 0.5 l/l/min, though this can be varied, and may be increased in the late stages of a fermentation to increase oxygen transfer when growth becomes thicker.

If a general investigation of a fermentation is being made, estimates of the respiration rates and values of the transfer coefficient K_{La} should be included. These investigations will be discussed in the next chapter.

A problem that arises in development work is the transfer of a new mutant or process from the laboratory to the plant. This may go smoothly or with difficulty, depending on the flexibility of the microbiological system and its ability to do equally well under the two sets of conditions. This subject will be discussed later, but some brief comments will be made at this stage.

Laboratory fermenters have particular characteristics in terms of mixing and oxygen transfer, and in the type of mycelium produced. New mutants and processes will be adapted to give optimal results under these conditions. Quite often, laboratory fermenters have automatic control of dissolved oxygen, and inoculum preparation may differ in laboratory and plant. Plant fermenters operate under higher air pressure due to the depth of the culture. Thus there are a number of limitations to contend with, and these are different from those in the laboratory equipment. As far as possible, laboratory fermenters should be adjusted to be as similar to the fermenters in the plant as possible. This so-called 'scale-down' problem is well recognised among workers in this field. One effect of this is the use of high-speed shakers, which give a closer approximation to the desired conditions. This matter is another aspect of the subject of 'scale up', which lies in the field of chemical engineering. For an account of some of the principles involved, see Lilly (1983). Although laboratory fermenters work well, the stirrers are much smaller in diameter, giving a Reynolds number:

$$Re = \frac{rpm \cdot D^2 \cdot density}{viscosity}$$

which is very much lower, if one compares stirrer diameters (D) in laboratory fermenters (e.g. 0.15 m) and in plant fermenters (e.g. 1.5 m) at, say, 700 and 120 rpm. The Reynolds number is an indicator of turbulence and mixing, and this could be an important factor in directing the course of the development of the microorganism.

To a considerable extent, the solution of the problem depends on the

Table 11.2. *Volume changes in a fermentation, on filtration*

Condition		Additions etc. (l)			Volumes (l)
Initial		medium	2.7		
		inoculum	0.3		3.0
Final	gains	feed etc.	0.3		
	losses	evaporation	0.2		
		samples	0.1		3.0
Nominal final volume					3.0
Final titre				10 g/l	
Actual volume		including air			3.2
Filtered volume			2.4		
		extra squeezing	0.2		
		or by			
		washing with	0.4		
Filtrate recovered,					
inclusive					3.0
Titre of total filtrate		becomes		8.7 g/l	

Example assumes a 3-l batch in a small fermenter.

management of the laboratory research programme. Those engaged in the field are usually well aware of the problem and can constantly make checks to avoid failure at plant level. This may be done by interspersing shaken-culture, stirred-culture, and larger-scale pilot-plant tests, or even by occasional trials in the main plant. This is all a matter of judgement and interdepartmental liaison and confidence.

Culture volumes

In laboratory work the main criterion of productivity is the titre of the antibiotic produced, i.e. the concentration in the medium, based on a filtered sample. In the plant, however, although the titre is a useful indicator, the criterion is the weight of product extractable from the batch. This depends on the efficiency of extraction, but also on the volume of filtrate obtained from the fermenter. This is less than the total culture volume and may be quite difficult to establish exactly. Laboratory workers should be aware of this problem because it can come as a surprise to the uninformed.

It is easier to visualise this in terms of a laboratory experiment in which the antibiotic is extracted, based on a 3-l culture in a small fermenter, assuming only two samples are withdrawn. Typical results for such a batch are summarised in Table 11.2. It is assumed that the filtrate from the last sample showed 10.0 g/l.

If the culture was removed and filtered and the filter-cake sucked as dry as possible, the filtrate would not reach 3.0 l. It might reach 2.3–2.4 l, or rather less. A small further quantity might be obtained by squeezing through rollers, to give about 2.5 l. In practice this extra filtrate would be obtained by washing the mycelium with a small volume of water, making the total 3.0 l, as shown in Table 11.2. owing to the dilution, the titre would be 8.7 g/l instead of 10.0 g/l. Assuming 80% recovery, the chemist carrying out the extraction would obtain 21 g of antibiotic, instead of the hoped for 24 g that might have been expected.

This loss of around 15% of the batch, due to filtration, also occurs in plant work. This is because the wet mycelium contains 65–75% moisture, so that if 40–50 of dry cells g/l are present, about 15% of the water in the medium is withdrawn, giving a concentrating effect, a situation very obvious in plant work.

In the plant this presents a statistical problem, which is usually dealt with by measuring the total culture volume by a convenient method, for example by weighing the hold-up vessel, and multiplying by a factor, e.g. 0.85, accepted in the light of experience.

11.3.3   Pipework systems in the fermentation plant

Three important systems of pipework are attached to the fermenters. One supplies sterile air, and another is used to transfer inoculum culture to the fermenter; sample withdrawal also comes into this category. The third system is used for the supply of antifoam and feeds and additions to the fermenter. The operation of these systems is highly important for success, especially as regards the avoidance of infection; therefore a brief account of them will be given. It will be realised that the system used in any plant is likely to be based on local opinion, and many variations will be observed in practice.

The sterile-air system

The elements of this system are sketched in Fig. 11.3. The blowers are usually of the turbine type, with a drive motor of several thousand horsepower. The main pipes are of large diameter, from which branches lead off to the individual fermenters. The main pipe is sub-divided by valves, and other valves are fitted in the lines leading to the fermenters. The pipework is designed to avoid the accumulation of water or waste at any point in the system. Air filters are fitted in the lines to the fermenters and may also be placed in the central main itself. There are various views on this subject. A special filter may be placed near the blower, to remove oil droplets. The air emerges from the pump at a high temperature and is not usually cooled. The volume of air may be about 1000 m³/min, i.e. 2.5 tonnes, at a pressure of 2–3 bars, as required by the fermenters. The compressors can be noisy, but this is avoided by careful design of the inlet.

The air filters may be packed with glass fibre or slag-wool formed into suitable blocks. A filter of this type might have a diameter of over 1 m, and

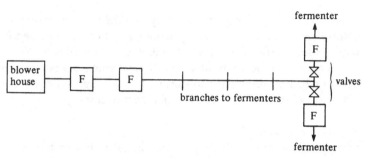

Fig. 11.3. Pipework for sterile air. F, filter.

a height of 1–1.5 m. Smaller filters, containing a ceramic filter unit or several units, are also used. In early models, difficulty was experienced in sealing the units to the base, and so leaks occurred, but this seems to have been overcome. Filters may be sterilised with steam under pressure, or by electric heating. The pipework has to be designed so that it can be steam sterilised and so that water cannot collect in it. The system for sterile-air supply is extensive and requires very careful design and construction. The valves in the pipe leading to each fermenter are doubled and arranged so that the fermenter can be sealed off from the main during preparation for a batch. During sterilisation, the link is re-sterilised. Typically, sterile-air mains will remain sterile continuously for 6–12 months between sterilisations. The testing of the sterility of the air is difficult; the fact that batches remain infection free is not conclusive, as single bacteria in the air may not be picked up in the fermenter. Specialised methods are used for testing the air. The main criterion has to be the good design of the system and the reliability of the filters, in terms of the absence of cracks or leaks, along with freedom from trouble in process operations.

Trouble with the sterile-air supply can arise from mistakes that cause a back pressure, so that culture flows back into the air system. This makes it necessary to clean and re-sterilise the system, which can be expensive as it often means closing down the plant temporarily. The most-common cause of this is a power failure, and fermentation plants may have to have an emergency system to allow the fermenter outlets to be shut off and the pressure maintained until the power is restored.

Culture transfer lines
A system of pipelines is provided for the transfer of inocula to the fermenters. This forms a branched system, with appropriate valves. This pipework is usually permanent, but in some cases detachable pipe units may be provided to cover different needs and to avoid the presence of unused pipes. It is customary to keep the pipes, when not in use, filled with steam under pressure, to avoid the possibility of infection.

The inoculation is said to be point when there is a considerable risk of infection. There is always a possibility that the pipes may retain old culture or wash water. It is also possible that there may be bends or dips in the pipes where liquid may accumulate, or there may be 'dead areas' which arise if a pipe is cut off and sealed, leaving a blank end, which can never be heated sufficiently to sterilise it. Although every effort may be made to avoid these dead ends, vigilance is necessary.

The feed-line networks

In a typical process, several types of feeds and additions may be involved. These fall into two types, relatively narrow-bore pipes to carry antifoam or special additions, added in small amounts, and wider pipes used for continuous feeding. With the first type, a quantity of solution may be prepared in a small tank, and it and the pipework may be sterilised so that the system can be used centrally over a long period. With feed, the solution is pumped to the fermenter through a heat exchanger that acts as a steriliser. In the simplest case, this consists of a length of large-diameter piping so designed that the solution is held within it, at a high temperature and pressure, for sufficient time for sterilisation, e.g. 30 min at 1 bar pressure. The pipework and steriliser is fitted with automatically controlled valves, so that if temperature or pressure are lost, the system will be shut down and sealed from the fermenter. These systems exist in a variety of forms, usually automated. In former times, the addition of carefully graded feeds were difficult to provide, but the introduction of the micro-processor has simplified the whole situation.

Some extra considerations apply in the case of additions to control pH and antifoam. In both cases, probes are available for measurement or detection. In the case of pH, however, the conditions of stirring and sterilisation are violent in large fermenters, and electrodes tend to fail. It is possible to replace pH electrodes during a batch, but the tendency is to base control on sampling. With foam control, at least three types of foaming are recognisable: (1) a very thin type of foam, which can occur very briefly at the start, is almost impossible to control and may be disregarded, (2) a thicker type of foam, which is readily controllable, at least by one of the modern antifoam agents, and (3) a type of thick foaming, when most of the batch turns into foam, is usually due to autolysis and is also very difficult to control; sometimes the airflow has to be reduced and stirring temporarily halted, though both processes are detrimental. Both pH changes and foaming are related to batch metabolism, and a principal aspect of control is the management of the batch so that additions are predictable and minimal so that out-of-control situations do not arise.

11.3.4   Sterilisation of plant equipment

In the laboratory, articles are sterilised by placing them in a steriliser and exposing them to steam for 20 min at 1 bar pressure, i.e. at 115 °C. They

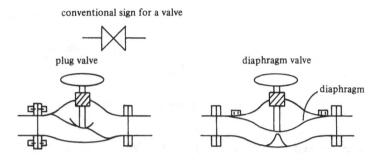

Fig. 11.4. Types of valves used for fermenters.

emerge sterile, and a feeling is often engendered that such treatment totally and automatically destroys all bacteria. That this is not actually so is easily shown by including among the articles a 5-l flask containing heavily contaminated broth. On incubation, the bacteria will grow again; this happens because the flask was not fully heated in the time allowed because of its size. Thus, we can say that by using a conventional period of 115 °C for 20 min, certain types of articles are freed from bacterial contamination, but that this only applies in the simple conventional case.

This point is important in plant work where there is no conventional situation, and in each circumstance, the particular time and temperature must be discovered and used. This is particularly so with a fermenter plus its pipework, where some parts are quickly heated, while others need a much longer period. For this reason heating at 120 or 125 °C for 30–45 min is commonly used, and sometimes longer heating is used, this suggesting a period of serious infection trouble in the past. There is a limit, because with long heating, the medium becomes dark, and then toxic.

In a fermentation plant, sterilisation routines are built up and tested in practice, so as to be usable with consistent success. The procedures are commonly automated, so that a fermenter and its associated equipment can be switched to the sterilisation cycle when required. When sterilisation fails, it usually means that some detail has been accidentally altered, leading to a danger spot that must be discovered and removed.

There are two points that need mention, the sterilisation of valves and pipe connections.

Sterilisation of valves
Types of valves commonly used are shown in Fig. 11.4. Ordinary plug or spade valves have a closing element that is screwed down with a screw and gland arrangement, which would not be sterilised by steaming, as part is external to the valve. For fermentation work, diaphragm valves are used (Fig. 11.4) in which the external mechanism is entirely separated from the internal pipe area. The special rubber diaphragms will last for a considerable time. The diaphragm is held in place by a metal bonnet

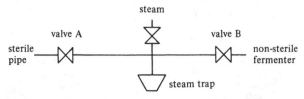

Fig. 11.5. Double-valve arrangement, for sterilisation of links.

which is bolted on to the top of the valve. While most valves are small, many valves with 15-cm or 20-cm bore are used; these are of considerable size and require a good deal of heat for sterilisation.

Sterilisation of pipe links
When a sterile pipeline is connected to a fermenter awaiting sterilisation, it is necessary to sterilise the link. This is done by using a pair of valves in tandem (Fig. 11.5). It is assumed that the left side of valve A is sterile. The intervening section is sterilised by passing steam into the link, with valve B open, while steam is passed into the fermenter. The steam trap passes condensed water, but not steam, so that the whole link and valves are sterilised. Alternatively, by opening valve A with B closed, the other side can be sterilised. Fermentation plants contain many of these double-valve systems for sterilisation; they make the pipework appear very complicated.

11.3.5　Fermentation shed staff
Different works show a variety of work systems, but the arrangements for the operations of the fermentation shed staff usually fall into two main groups, shift workers who run the fermenters and provide 24-h cover, and day workers who do supporting work. Shift workers work a week of 35–38 h, and there are two or three shifts per day, according to custom. There are therefore usually five teams: two or three at work, and the remainder having rest-days or longer breaks, the shift rota being planned over several weeks. The works staff is thus much larger than appears at first sight, and, if the researcher has become accustomed to one of the teams, it can be disconcerting when it disappears for several weeks. Considerable alterations to schedules occur at holiday times.

The day workers carry out a wide range of duties. These include the preparation of batches of materials for the fermentations, receipt of deliveries, warehousing, maintenance of stores, and cleaning, as well as looking after the clothing and the laundry arrangements. Shift workers have usually received some advanced education and are also trained within the company.

The shed is under the charge of a manager with a number of assistants. There is usually a great deal to do, for example overseeing the current manufacturing programme, and preparing future work schedules, along with arranging for maintenance and repair work and ordering supplies, together with general supervising. A good deal of work arises from looking after the staff and seeing to their personal requirements, and arranging cover when staff are sick or on leave. There is little time to act as nurse to the visiting researcher.

11.3.6   Fermentation control and the use of computers
Introduction
As would be expected, when a batch is started, the procedure follows a carefully planned system. Each stage is designed to give optimal results, while relying on carefully controlled procedures. These procedures involve the preparation and sterilisation of the media, and the control of the fermentation at each stage, including such factors as fermentation temperature, air pressure, and flow rate, together with planned feeds and additions. During all stages of the batch, careful records are kept to ensure that the process is closely in line with the planned procedure. As mentioned, records were formerly based on instrument recorder charts and manual listing. More recently, the instrumentation and recording has been largely computerised and centralised in a control room.

During the overall fermentation plan (Table 11.1), the control of the short pre-production stages presents few problems, but during the long production fermentation, the control methods may become more elaborate. Although batches may be supposed to be identical, there are often slight variations in the rate of progress, so that the feed plan may have to be adjusted to give the best results. This requires daily or 12-hourly (or more often) estimates of the state of the batch. In the laboratory, automatic analysers may be used, but in the plant, the analyses are usually manual and are carried out, as required, by the process workers, a small laboratory being attached to the control room for the purpose. Spot tests are used for factors such as pH, residual sugar in the medium, growth by packed cell volume, colour and odour, and perhaps phosphate, ammonia, and the antibiotic itself. Sugar (as glucose, after hydrolysis) can be measured using tablets or test papers used by diabetics, and ammonia can be measured by adding alkali to a sample and drawing air through the solution, the ammonia being trapped in dilute acid and estimated by back-titration. The assay of the antibiotic may require the help of a specialist. The results of these quick tests may be approximate, but they enable a skilled worker to make a good estimate of the state of the batch, and then to adjust the feeds and other conditions in an optimal manner. Success depends on experience and on an understanding of the way microorganisms react, and workers differ in the degree of success they achieve. The success of this approach depends on the fact that all the batches are the same (for a given antibiotic). In the laboratory, the batches tend to vary as different conditions are tested.

Two points require comment. The total number of analyses made per shift is probably small, and the provision of a shift analyst would not be justified. In addition, automated apparatus for analysis is usually unnecessary, since, for the data required, it would be expensive and would require careful maintenance and oversight. The other point is that an immediate result is needed, on which to base action. Control is based on the variation of the factor or factors measured, and figures some hours old, needing extrapolation, would be useless. The measurement of antibiotic is less critical, as assays once or twice a day will give the slope sufficiently well, and this can be compared with expectations as required. The analyses are for immediate practical use; later contemplation of them is secondary.

Computer control of plant operations
The whole fermentation process, from medium make-up through to harvesting, requires a great deal of work and much attention to careful control and monitoring. It is natural that much effort is put into the use of computers for this purpose. Although computers are widely employed, the subject is changing and developing continually, and this will continue into the future.
The computer system might provide for the following functions.

(a) Issue of instructions for batches, and provision of details for medium preparation etc.
(b) During medium make-up, the checking of the addition of the main components to the mixing vessel; this checking is done by means of a load cell.
(c) Conduct of sterilisation.
(d) Set up controls and details for batch operation, e.g. temperature, airflow, feed profile, etc.
(e) Record all details in memory and by print-out.
(f) In the event of a breakdown, to issue alarms and re-set valves to ensure safety.
(g) When necessary, information, analyses, etc., to be entered by keyboard.
(h) Although the computer could provide data on which the feed profile might be modified automatically, decisions would be made by the supervisor or manager.
(i) At the end of the fermentation, the computer could discharge the culture for extraction, wash down the fermenter, and prepare for the next batch.

Commenting on this list, a large industrial firm agreed that the computer could do all these things, but not all these facilities were used in their plant. There are many reasons for this, one being the management's preference for a more flexible system of operation.

The earlier control rooms tended to be complex, with wall displays of the plant, and desks with miniature gauges and switches to provide control. The modern trend is towards greater simplification and minimal detail (Society of Chemical Industry, 1986). The plant is usually divided into areas, for example a fermenter and its supporting equipment, each monitored by a micro-processor linked to the main computers, which can be used directly in the event of a breakdown.

Information collected from instruments is on pressure, temperature, stirring, aeration rates, etc., along with feed additions and analytical data, some of which may be obtained by the controller himself. Thus, at given intervals, the computer has a comprehensive picture of the situation. It will be realised that at a given time, say 72 h, all these values will, with a normal batch, have particular values. Typical measurements may include feed added, pH, alkali used for pH control, ammonia and other medium constituents, organic and inorganic, cell concentration, antibiotic production, and others. If these figures vary from the normal levels, then the fermentation can be regarded as abnormal, to varying degrees. Initially the data would be presented in figures (e.g. Table 8.2). This is not very helpful to a busy controller, and the modern tendency is to use an interactive expert system (Branch, 1986) to present the position in words, for example 'normal', 'slightly abnormal', 'requires adjustment', or 'out of control: alert', the latter being emphasised by flashing the words. The main visual display unit (VDU) could then present the position of all the fermenters, 20 or more, as fermenter numbers, batch and product numbers, and age, and then it could present a comment on the state of the batch. If a batch moved away from normal, the supervisor could call it onto another VDU and obtain several pages of information and advice, in increasing levels of detail. This is a developing area, and is obviously of importance in connection with the treatment of batch fluctuations, to be discussed in Chapter 13. This system will also deal with technical faults and mechanical breakdowns.

The extent to which computers are used varies between plants. In some cases all the valves and parameters would be set via the computer. The conversion of an old but effective plant from manual to fully automated control would be very expensive, and, in such cases, the computer would be used for recording and programming the feed systems. This would involve much interaction between computer and manual control. It is unlikely that the degree of computerisation achieved in chemical plants could be reached in fermentation sheds, especially because of the skill needed in applying analytical data in controlling the process, which relies so much on the judgement of the experienced staff.

A most-serious problem is caused by an electrical power failure, which can cause widespread trouble. The loss of pressure in the air mains can cause the flow of culture between the fermenters and into the filters if

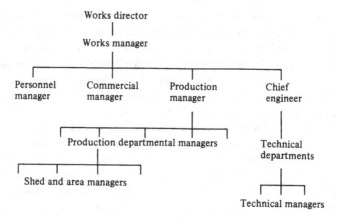

Fig. 11.6. Factory organisation.

action is not taken at once to close down the fermenters and apply an emergency input of air. Computer failure causes trouble, but the plant can continue to be operated by the micro-processors in each area, together with some manual control.

11.4   The organisation of the antibiotics factory
11.4.1   The management system

There is much variation in the organisation of antibiotics factories, depending on their size and their place in the firm's organisation, but a common outline can be observed, as indicated in Fig. 11.6. The various managers would have assistant managers to deal with different aspects of their work. The personnel manager would deal with staff matters, training, and the like, the commercial manager would deal with costing and purchasing, while the chief engineer would be in charge of a wide range of daily and long-term problems and projects. There is usually a production manager responsible for the various branches of works activity, such as fermentation, extraction, the analytical services, special products, and research, though research might be administered in a different way. The works director (or works manager) would provide liaison with the firm's directorate. The works is likely to be turning over large sums of money, and the administration is of great practical importance, since if mistakes are made, considerable problems can arise.

To the researcher, this organisation may seem remote, but it is important to know who is who and to be aware of the managers to whom the research is relevant. It is also important to know the correct routes to get help and advice. Managers tend to be jealous about their departments, so it is best to follow the rules. Works commonly work

Table 11.3. *Subdivision of costs*

(1)	Cost of materials and services
(2)	Cost of wages and salaries
(3)	Overheads

through committees, and the senior people are usually aware of what is going on in different areas of work. This generally shared knowledge is a feature of works life and can be a very helpful factor in research.

A considerable part of management's time is taken up with planning future production. This takes place in conjunction with the firm's headquarters, especially with the sales department and its various planning groups. In this process the next year's manufacturing plan and costings are subject to critical scrutiny. Details of this may not be known to individual researchers, but it makes the reliability of research predictions of great importance. It is therefore useful if the researcher has some knowledge of the economics of manufacture and is aware of the firm's thinking on the subject.

11.4.2 Fermentation economics

Only a brief and simplified account of this subject will be given here. There are differences in the way firms deal with the subject, and the costs of fuel and materials can vary from one time to another, so that to attempt to go into detail could be erroneous or misleading. A fuller discussion is provided by Stowell & Bateson (1983).

The costs of production in the fermentation plant can be divided into three main areas, as shown in Table 11.3. The first two of these are readily explicable, the first consisting of nutrients and materials used for plant maintenance etc., together with services such as water, electricity, and fuel. These service costs are very large, being measured in millions of pounds. The second area, salaries and wages, is clear enough.

The subject of overheads is more complex. Overheads cover the repayment of the building of the plant and of interest on loans, local and central taxation, plus works costs such as roads, painting, etc., and charges from other departments. Overheads also include the firm's charges for the directorate, research, and other factors, which can amount to a goodly sum.

Owing to differences in the way different firms calculate amounts, the ratio between the three items varies, but it is reasonable to assume that the three are about equal.

In planning each year's output, the parties concerned agree upon a level of production for each product, plus the cost per gram or kilogram as it leaves the works, referred to as the normal or standard cost. These evaluations provide the targets for the next year.

During production, the antibiotic is produced by fermentation and then extracted and stored in the warehouse. It can then be passed to the pharmaceutical plant at the normal cost, or sold with an appropriate profit. The pharmaceutical material can then be sold to a wholesaler, at a profit, and the wholesaler will sell it onwards for use. An idea of costs, in late 1984, can be obtained for penicillin. Industrial workers have quoted a price of £12/kg, i.e. 1.2p/g. Potassium penicillin-V was quoted for sale in New York at 2.5¢/g, equivalent to about 1.8p/g, suggesting some addition for the wholesaler.

The sub-division of costs in Table 11.3 is rough and ready, but it suggests the following:

(a) The contribution of single items to costs is small, so that the use of less of a single item will have little effect on the total cost of the antibiotic.

(b) An increase in output from the same materials should lower the cost per gram.

(c) The costs mentioned relate to the works internal budget. As the products move to the pharmaceuticals plant, to the wholesaler, and to the pharmacy, additions to the price take place, part of which is profit. The ultimate sales price will be a proportion of the price charged, so that the value of the final product is an index of the profit obtained. Taking the prices of different types of penicillin, the literature gives the following.

Penicillin (ex works)   1.2p/g
Penicillin tablets   4.0p/g
Semi-synthetic penicillin (ampicillin)   15p/g

It will be seen that as the penicillin leaves the fermentation plant, the extra work put in increases the cost, but it also increases the profit per gram produced. There is therefore a desire to sell a highly developed product instead of the raw material. The minute contribution of the cost of a high-technology product may suggest the advantage of purchase of raw material, instead of manufacture. Penicillin is a mass-produced antibiotic, and a cheap price is essential. Manufacturers prefer to sell their own novel products where profitability is easier to achieve.

(d) It is often advisable to break down the cost in Table 11.3 in more detail, by considering how expenses increase with time. Thus the cleaning and preparation of the plant, the medium, and the inoculum produce a large immediate cost, after which there are daily costs for salaries, power, etc. The breakdown of costs is valuable in assessing the most-economic length of the fermentation.

In manufacture, there is considerable use of flexible costing. Thus a product may be made in small amounts, rather expensively, but be a useful sales attraction. Some of its costs of manufacture may be loaded onto a large-scale, profitable product, since it can be argued that if the minor product was abandoned, part of the plant would be empty and the staff underemployed.

Although the subject of costs may not be of great importance to a scientist engaged in process development, some knowledge of the principles is useful. The major factors in manufacture are output and costs, and it is impossible to ignore them when considering practical process development.

11.4.3   The antibiotics factory as a community

While research departments often consist of groups who know each other well, there are often people in the department one never meets and of whom one may never even hear. In the works, however, where people have worked together for years, there is much more sense of community. It is worthwhile for an incomer to recognise this pattern, with all its cross-relationships. If the researcher has arrived to help with a difficulty, it is an affair in which everybody is involved.

The situation can have several effects. On the one hand there is a desire to help, and there is also a desire to see what happens. There may also be a fear that the newcomer may try to boost his importance by blaming or criticising the local folk, and he is therefore to be regarded with suspicion, especially if he sneaks about when the supervisor is not looking. If the right course is steered, the involvement can be an enjoyable period of life, with many valuable contacts for the future.

11.5   The industrial pilot plant

In an industrial plant, development work should be unnecessary, as only well-designed and reliable processes are operated. In practice, a good deal of work may be needed, mainly to check strains and materials and to solve local problems.

The position in different factories varies. Some, being related to a large central organisation, possibly abroad, will have a few fast shakers and assistance from the local analytical laboratory with which to make routine tests, major tasks being performed at the central establishment. In other cases, the research pilot plant may be in the works, like the one illustrated in Chapter 7, and will be well equipped and run by a specialist staff, who conduct basic research on the site. Thus researchers becoming involved with plant problems may simply walk across the yard, or they may come from a distance into unfamiliar circumstances.

12 Process development in the fermentation plant

12.1 Introduction

Development work in the plant is needed for a number of reasons. These may be the need to introduce a new process developed in the laboratory, the need to improve existing plant processes and to correct faults, and the need to deal with problems like infection. Constant attention is needed to hold an existing high standard of working, as results may drift downwards over a long period. There may be times when it is desired to reduce the rate of production, temporarily, and an economical process may be needed to make this possible. The two serious problems that sometimes arise, infection and yield fluctuation, are discussed in Chapter 13, where methods for the study of plant batches are also considered.

This subject has been discussed in a number of papers, for example Queener & Swartz (1979), Küenzi & Auden (1983), and in general by Vandamme (1984). These accounts tend to stress the difficulty and complexity of the subject. This is often the case, especially with highly developed processes. In the earlier stages this is often less difficult. With penicillin, for example, the early processes worked quite well in the plant, though infection and reproducibility presented greater problems. Often the initial difficulty is to get good growth in the inoculum; this difficulty can be overcome after a certain amount of experimentation. As the process is developed, problems such as those described in Chapters 5 and 6 become more apparent. As production increases and the steps in progress become less, the critical factors become more important, and experimental work becomes more difficult to interpret.

In theory, plant fermentations should behave as laboratory ones do, and the various ideas about how laboratory fermentations work should also be transferable, although the parameters might be different, and the conditions might be less easy to define due to differences in the equipment. In practice, the situation is not so simple. There are also differences in approach between laboratory and plant workers, and less experimental data is available. Plant workers may also be unenthusiastic unless they are convinced of the likelihood of success. Analytical facilities may also differ. If the research laboratory is nearby, the situation is convenient. If it is at a distance, the investigator will have to do the best he can. One effect of this is that the laboratory worker makes use of a set of ideas, different from those among the plant team, who base their ideas on different ideas and other types of measurements. This pattern is

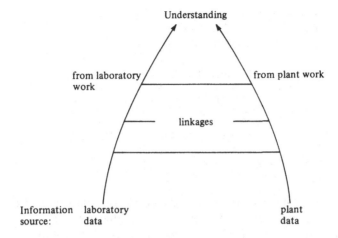

Fig. 12.1. Development of an understanding of a fermentation.

illustrated in Fig. 12.1. It may be necessary for the process developer to make special tests in the laboratory to be able to appreciate both systems, and to avoid the appearance of being a *deus ex machina*. The collection of data in the plant is discussed in Chapter 13.

The subject of process development will be discussed here from the point of view of an experienced laboratory worker who is not very familiar with works conditions, which it is necessary to become accustomed to. This makes it easier to bring out the problems likely to be encountered, and how they can be dealt with. Each worker sees the subject in his or her own way and must choose the best approach to the task.

12.2   Plant development: trials of new processes

12.2.1   Planning the trials

Laboratory work is the starting point, providing a suggestion for improving plant output. This may follow the isolation of a new mutant, or the development of a new fermentation process. This would lead, in turn, to a proposal that a trial should be made, and agreement that the work be put in hand.

The first stage is to prepare an account of the proposals. This account should contain the relevant experimental data and should present details of the test to be carried out. Although the methods to be followed will be worked out in conjunction with plant management, it is important to convey conviction as to the reliability of the basis of the proposals, and to be clear about the details to be followed. From experience, it can be said that the amount of detail required by the plant management is likely to depend on previous experience of the antibiotic process concerned. If

Table 12.1. *Prediction of number of
replicates needed, in relation to the
expected increase in yield*

Expected increase %	Number of replicates[a]		
	15% SE	10% SE	7.5% SE
25	3.4	2.1	1.6
15	7.7	4.0	2.7
7.5	27.6	12.8	7.7

[a] For $P = 0.1$

trials have previously gone well and the new data looks promising, there
will be anxiety to go ahead. If there has been difficulty in the past,
enthusiasm will be less. It is always unwise to proceed if there is any
vagueness or uncertainty over the methods and results. The statistical
basis for the trial should be considered (next section). It will be realised
that the success of the trial depends on the success of scaling up from
laboratory to plant, and it is usually essential that the yield not be below
normal.

When trying a new process, it is customary to carry out a trial batch. If
this works well then more will be run until the position becomes clear. The
numbers required will usually be based on a statistical analysis of the
results, as they appear. Success may be judged on the basis of the titre
obtained, but it usually includes the results of extraction and isolation
work; also, if the fermentation time has been extended, the extra cost of
this will have to be taken into account.

12.2.2 *Statistical considerations in planning*

It is worth considering the statistical aspect of plant trials. Relevant
information on this subject will be found in the textbooks. This makes it
possible to calculate the number of tests likely to be needed, based on a
knowledge of the standard error (SE, %) obtained from a number of
normal batches. For example, the SE % may be 10%, based on the
average of ten standard batches. The value of t from 9 degrees of freedom
is then 1.83 (P (probability coefficient) $= 0.10$) and 2.26 ($P = 0.05$),
from tables. The number of degrees of freedom in a test, expecting an
increase of D%, compared with the standard method, is then:

$$n = \left(\frac{t \cdot \sqrt{2} \cdot SE}{D}\right)^2$$

so that the number of replicates required will be $n + 1$.

The values for the numbers of replicates required for different values of
SE and D are given in Table 12.1, based on $P = 0.1$, a level of significance

sufficient to indicate that further trials are justified. For $P = 0.05$, 50% more replicates would be required.

Table 12.1 throws considerable light on the problem of plant trials and the demands arising when only small advances are under consideration. This is also important practically with regard to the time likely to be needed to carry out a large number of tests. The calculations relate also to laboratory work. They show why so many tests are needed in the later stages of process improvement, when advances are around 10%. They also show why there is so much interest in adjusting laboratory conditions to resemble the plant, thus avoiding the need for extensive plant trials.

12.2.3　Conduct of the trials

The trials should be planned in detail. In a typical plant process, a batch starts from a slope and passes through several pre-production stages before the main batch commences. If a new mutant is being introduced, it should be tested throughout all these stages, before the production trial, to make sure that it grows satisfactorily. It is important that the research worker follows all these stages of the process to make sure that all is well and to make a comparison with laboratory results and with the behaviour of the standard process. Samples from these stages should be transferred to the laboratory for production tests in shaken or, preferably, stirred culture. Morphological examination and cell concentration measurements should be carried out. During the production stage, at least some data on respiration rates and dissolved oxygen should be collected. It is advisable to carry out a range of tests on the early test batches, and to do some also on standard batches, since if the programme is stopped, the opportunity will be lost with it. This data can be of value in research, when the results are reviewed. It may be possible to obtain only a few results per batch, but this will be well worthwhile. This follow-up work may be demanding, requiring observations at night, but round-the-clock data collection gives the clearest picture during critical stages. Adequate assays of the antibiotic concentrations should also be obtained. All details should be carefully noted.

Although the fermentation work will be conducted by plant staff, the research worker should maintain close contact on the site, so that there is no doubt about the way the fermentations went during all the stages of the process. The liaison with plant colleagues is helpful, and it makes direct comparisons with laboratory fermentations much easier.

12.2.4　Assessment of results and future action

If the initial batch suggests that it is safe to proceed, several further batches will be carried out to build up sufficient data for a statistical check on the experiment. The results may then show results that are equal or better than standard, or that are worse, the extent of the change being expressed as a percentage. The results of the experiment can then be judged in terms of the expectations:

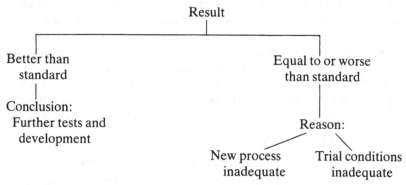

The meaning of 'better than standard' depends on expectations and the state of development. It could be 25–100% in the early stages of development; later on, 10–15% might be thought good enough. If there is no advance it may be that the new process is of too little advantage, or that trial conditions were unsuitable. In either case, it is necessary to consider carefully whether it is worth continuing with the new mutant or process in the hope of success, or whether it is better to continue with laboratory work until a larger advantage is obtained. It can be damaging to continue with plant trials when success seems unlikely.

An example of an unsuccessful test is given in Table 12.2, based on old records. It shows the way in which the advantage obtained in initial laboratory trials can fall away as conditions change. The advantage shown in stirred fermenters, which was sufficient to be of interest commercially and would have been expected to show up in the plant, failed to carry through on this occasion.

When the results are disappointing, the decision about future action depends on the circumstances. Much will depend on the observations made during the tests, and on the analytical data. These might suggest the type of growth patterns obtained in the plant throughout all the stages was not optimal, so that work on this aspect is needed. This would require work in large pilot-plant fermenters to bring out the details and the possibility of an improvement. Very much depends on how well the process is understood and the reliability of predictions of the success of transfer from laboratory to plant.

12.2.5   Fine tuning with a highly developed process

Characteristically, the earlier stages of development are relatively easy, with the difficulty increasing as production increases. As the stage of maximal yields is reached, the work increases greatly in complexity, especially as the degree of advance become less, and testing becomes

Table 12.2. *Example of test of new process*

Type of test	Replication	Average results (relative units)	
		standard	new
Shaken flasks	24 flasks	7.5	11.5
Stirred fermenters	2 tests, 3 replicates	8.3	10.3
Plant	6–7 replicates	9.3	8.8

Standard error, ± 10% of mean.

more difficult. An example from this area of work has been given by Küenzi & Auden (1983), who stress the problem produced by the different behaviour shown in flasks, stirred fermenters, and the plant, which makes experimental planning difficult. They also stress the importance of examining as many variables as possible during trials, starting with the shaken flasks. Small differences can indicate the strengths and weaknesses of the strains and the best method to avoid the difficulties they produce.

These authors give the results of development work based on a mutant producing cephalosporin C; this work gave an increase of 10% in shaken flasks. Results in pilot-plant fermenters, adjusted to resemble large fermenters as regards their fermentation characteristics, are shown in Table 12.3. Values are expressed as a percentage of the control. The mutant gave a lower yield in the fermenters, compared to the standard method, but by changing the system in a number of ways, an increase in titre of 21% was obtained, and about 11% in productivity, i.e. in economic terms, probably taking into account some extension of the fermentation time. A development of this kind exhibits a great deal of skill on the part of the workers, together with much time required in the pilot plant. It is interesting to see physical factors involved in the work. The use of temperature to control the rate of growth goes back a long way, historically, in fermentation work. Küenzi & Auden stress the importance of the ability to decide when a particular line of development should be broken off because it shows too little promise.

In discussing this highly sophisticated work, these authors stress that the factors involved in increased yields are not usually additive, and that it would be difficult to model them adequately. All the same, it is likely that some kinds of informal models are developed to at least give a feeling of how the systems work and what the limitations are, to help in planning, and to correlate the results of different experiments. They also recommend the use of extensive analyses of factors that change during the

Table 12.3. *Improvement of cephalosporin C fermentations*

Step	Parameter adjusted	Productivity (% of control)	Max. titre (% of control)
0	standard conditions	97	95
1	N-source, temperature, phosphate	98	103
2	N-source	104	100
3	pH, head pressure in fermenter	107	115
4	N-source, carbon feed	111	121

From Küenzi & Auden (1983).

fermentation, as a means of characterising the conditions in different types of fermenter. This is a most useful experimental concept.

Each experimenter has to base his or her work in some such way on experience. Skill in planning, in finding bases, in developing a feeling for the way individual fermentations work, and in acquiring images or models of the processes are essential features of development research; these skills should be cultivated and regarded as an important and positive part of the work. Each case must be investigated on its own merits, and action must be taken in accordance with the demands of the situation. With different antibiotics, the relation between the physiology and biochemistry of the cells and the biosynthetic effect is probably unique, rather than part of a quite general pattern.

13 Two plant problems: infection and variations in the level of production

Infection and yield variations can cause serious problems in production work. In the early days of the antibiotics industry, infection was often a most-serious problem, sometimes halting production for months at a time. The situation greatly improved after several years' hard work, and plants now work over long periods without trouble. Infection can occasionally break out, and a brief description of the problems it creates is therefore useful.

Outbreaks of groups of low-yielding batches, lasting for periods of time, can also cause trouble. These outbreaks may be of two kinds. Firstly there are relatively small drops in yields (15–25%), probably caused by variations in technique. Secondly, very severe falls in output, to 50%, sometimes less, associated with changed metabolism, for which there is no obvious reason.

These two problems, of infection and yield variation, are difficult to deal with. A team effort between engineers and plant staff is usually needed, a microbiologist being often called in to provide an extra pair of eyes and hands, since it usually happens that the local people find the cure. The two problems, however, are often related, since falls in yield may be due to infection, and it may be necessary to decide which.

13.1 The problem of infection
13.1.1 The nature of infection

Infection arises from the contamination of the batches with invading microorganisms, usually bacteria. Infection may be at low or high level. The first may have little or no effect, while with a heavy infection there are serious changes in appearance, and the culture has to be discarded. In most cases, the infection is relatively low, but it is noticeable, has some effect on production, and can be confirmed by testing. With some slight infections, the main batch may seem little affected, but on harvesting and filtration, there is a considerable loss of product. In any case, infection leads to uncertainty, which is most harmful to steady production and process development.

While infection is sometimes caused by fungi or streptomycetes, it is usually caused by bacteria or yeasts. The bacteria are often gram-negative rods of a type occurring in natural waters (e.g. *Aeromonas, Alkaligenes,*

181

and the like, *Achromobacterium*, and sometimes Pseudomonads). These are not always easily recognised by microbiologists who are unfamiliar with them. Many grow only at 20–25 °C or below, so they will be missed on incubation at 30–37 °C. Occasionally cocci or spore-bearers may appear.

The type of organism involved can give an indication of the source. Infection with spore-bearers suggests inadequate heating, though non-sporing bacteria may also survive a considerable degree of heat. The bacteria isolated may represent the population of the plant, in dust etc., and it may be worth making tests to check this point.

Infection can be detected in several ways, and routine tests are carried out on plant samples, using methods adapted to the process in question. These tests may include the following.

(a) Direct inspection of the culture for turbidity of the supernatant and an unusual odour.

(b) Microscopic examination. For this the writer prefers unstained preparations, since this enables motility to be observed.

(c) Culture tests. With obvious infection, the addition of a loopful of medium to slopes or broth, followed by incubation at 25 °C, will bring out growth. With suspected trace infections, larger amounts should be used, for example 5 ml may be added to production medium in a shaken flask, which is then incubated on the shaker and examined both for infection and production.

In difficult cases, careful planning of the infection tests becomes necessary, so as to take into account all the circumstances of the case.

Infection can also be a problem in laboratory work, and it may not always be easy to solve. It is usually possible, though, to attack it directly by dismantling the equipment. This is followed by careful reassembly and sterilisation. The laboratory fermenter may then be filled with nutrient broth and incubated. Fermentation plants are so large and complex that this cannot be done, and a test using broth would be expensive. The search for a fault requires a careful examination of plant and procedures, and it may take a considerable time.

Serious infection problems are most harmful to morale, and they can lead to severe precautions to prevent contamination. These may involve prolonged sterilisation at high temperatures, which reduces the productivity of the cultures because the medium is rendered toxic.

13.1.2   Sources of infection in the plant

In modern times plants are usually built by specialist firms and are designed to avoid infection. This should eliminate the problem, but compromises often have to be made, both in design and in plant operation, and these compromises make contamination possible. Table 13.1 summarises some possible causes of infection. A consideration of

Table 13.1. *Possible sources of infection*

(1)	Leaks and other weaknesses in fermenters and pipework
(2)	Inadequate sterilisation procedures
(3)	Areas that are difficult to sterilise due to design faults or unsuitable modifications, or to dirty operating conditions
(4)	By accidental connection of non-sterile equipment to the fermentation system
(5)	From mal-operation of the sterile-air system
(6)	Problems with transfer lines used for inoculation and provision of feeds
(7)	Weaknesses in operational procedures, which may arise from process changes during development
(8)	Infection may arise at the point when seed is introduced to start the culture

these points suggests areas for examination and evaluation, where inspections and tests should be made so as to clarify the situation.

In considering an infection problem, a good deal turns on where the infection appears, for example in the inoculum stages, or early or late in the fermentation. If it appears very late, it must have arisen in the main fermentation itself. In general, operational mistakes cause heavy infection, with almost immediate collapse of production.

As regards leakages due to seepage, pinholes, and the like, these are usually covered by routine maintenance checks and repairs, and they can be held in check. They can be more dangerous in old plants, when corrosion or cracking and other faults start to appear, and they require repairs. This applies also to the sterile-air system. The mains water may be at a very high pressure at times (10 bar), and this can force non-sterile water from cooling coils into the batch.

While operational routines are usually carefully planned and as safe as possible, modifications involving risks can become customary and are often started with the best of intentions.

13.1.3 Sterilisation failures

Sterilisation failures are of two main kinds.

(a) The sterilisation of large plant items is difficult because of their complexity. The fermenters, mechanical seals, and ancillary equipment such as heat-exchangers etc. have to be sterilised with the valves (to the exterior) open, using the double-valve system previously described. There may be a number of these items. The overall heating of the fermenter must allow for these attachments. As mentioned in Chapter 3, the effect of heat is to produce killing exponentially with time, i.e. for any equipment the necessary time and temperature must be determined by experience. While this will allow a margin for error, the possibility for a failure must be taken into account at one point or another. Sterilisation at 125 °C for 45 min seems adequate for most purposes.

(b) The other possibility is that some part of the plant may be almost impossible to sterilise. This can occur in pipe sections where water may accumulate, or in dead ends or flanges for the introduction of instrument probes. These can become filled with mycelium that is never properly heated. It is also possible that there are places in the fermenters where a mass of mycelium can build up, in which bacteria are protected by the presence of protein or fat. These accumulations are usually avoided in the design, but they may arise in the course of modifications.

Sterile-air systems are usually carefully designed and are, if well maintained, satisfactory. As a rule, the main air-supply network is sterilised periodically. Although there is a tendency to suspect the sterile-air system, it usually turns out to be in order. The testing of the air requires special techniques and special apparatus, which is usually available on manufacturing sites.

13.1.4   Investigation of infection

The control-chart approach, described below, will bring out certain features of the infection situation. Plotting can be based on production figures when low yields correspond to infection, or batches can be plotted as infected or not infected. This may show several types of situations. Often it is normal for a few batches to be infected (2–5%). The sudden appearance of a large number of infections implies a change in circumstances that may involve some fermenters but not others. Another situation would be the occurrence of groups of infected batches, each lasting for a limited period. The time or stage when infection appeared is also important.

Having established some sort of rationale, it is necessary to look back into the records to see if the outbreak of infection is associated with any particular event. This search must go back to the seed-culture area. If any signs of an association can be found, then it must be examined in more detail.

If infection seems to break out at a particular date, it suggests that a significant change in circumstances must have occurred at that time. This might be as follows.

(a) A change in the master culture, or in some aspect of the pre-production stages.

(b) A change in technique in the fermentation process. This could involve a wide range of activities.

(c) That the infection has followed engineering work done on the plant, the effect showing up a few days later. This may not be easy to track down, because engineering maintenance work goes on all the time, so that infection following one of the jobs done might not be obvious.

As mentioned, it is difficult for a researcher to detect the cause of infection when the plant staff have already spent a good deal of time on the work and have been unsuccessful. In these circumstances it is often worthwhile inspecting the plant, preferably accompanied by a staff member, to look for possible weaknesses from a fresh standpoint. This could be done during sterilisation, or when routine aseptic operations are in progress. During sterilisation, temperatures can be checked with heat-sensitive crayons or in other ways. Attention should be given to the general standards of skill of the operators and the cleanliness of the operation. In this way, estimates of risk can be made. It is on estimates of risk that a conclusion may have to be reached. The examination of an antibiotics plant is a complicated operation, really requiring engineering training. It is sometimes possible for a microbiologist who does not accept that a layout is correct because it agrees with the blueprint to see that some parts of the equipment are over-complicated and perhaps unsafe against infection.

In the end, the questions may turn out to be a matter of opinion. Are the plant and techniques sufficiently safe? Is an undetected mistake likely to be occurring? Can tests be made that will clear up these three aspects? Often the answer is a matter of logic, rather than of testing alone.

13.2   Batch-to-batch variation and the problem of falling production

Under good conditions, plant fermentations usually work steadily, with a standard error of about 10% of the results. At times, outbreaks of low-yielding batches can occur. These are of two types, small and large fluctuations from normal. The position is illustrated in Fig. 13.1. Line 1 shows the expected norm, line 2 shows end retardation of production, while line 3 shows a low-yielding batch, though the effect is not severe. Lines 4 and 5 can be regarded as representing severe fluctuations from normal. In the case of lines 2 and 3, the behaviour of the batches could be detected by antibiotic assays, and it would probably be desirable to harvest them early to save the expense of the last 2 or 3 days with low productivity. With the severely affected batches, it would be necessary to detect them as early as possible, and to take action to recover at least some product from them to cover works expenses. The first type of variation (Fig. 13.1, lines 1 and 2) often arises from minor variations in batch operation, which are unavoidable in works practice, or from small

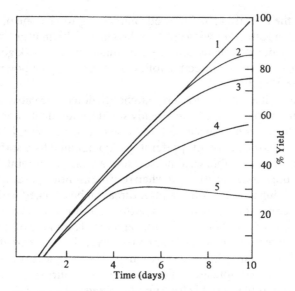

Fig. 13.1. Patterns of production. Curves: 1, standard; 2, end retardation; 3, low
yield; 4, severe fluctuation; 5, batch failure.

changes in the process, introduced for convenience, that have an
unexpected effect. Severe fluctuations (Fig. 13.1, lines 4 and 5) present a
more difficult problem. They are often accompanied by changes in the
patterns of growth and metabolism, indicating a major disturbance to the
system. They are recognisable to those familiar with the system, and
suggest an instability in cell regulation that is liable to go out of control.
As a matter of convenience, the first types of behaviour will be dealt with
in the present section, and the problem of severe fluctuations will be dealt
with in Section 13.3.

In dealing with these problems, there is a need to establish methods for
recognising the state of affairs as early as possible (diagnosis) so as to
work out a plan for future action, if necessary (treatment). This makes
great demands on all concerned.

The situation resembles that of doctor and patient. The doctor seeks
symptoms that form a pattern leading to diagnosis. This may suggest a
cure or may call for the aid of a specialist. The diagnosis depends on the
doctor possessing mental images of the association between tests and
diagnosis, and these images are learnt and then developed systematically
during the daily round. A systematic approach of this type must be
cultivated in development work, and it is particularly relevant to plant
problems. The different sorts of information available in laboratory and
plant (cf. Fig. 12.1) must be included in this learning process.

It will be realised that the main contributors to the solution of this problem (as with infection) are likely to be the plant staff, who have a greater instinctive understanding of the subject. The researcher's contribution is mainly to try to achieve a more rigid understanding of the situation, so as to improve diagnosis and to design the problem out of the fermentation.

It should be added that yield fluctuations can cease unexpectedly, which makes their study more difficult than ever. On starting an investigation, it is therefore advisable to get some quick data from the plant by sampling several batches at different ages, and by making some simple tests, such as pH, packed cell volume, microscopic appearance, titre, and any other tests that can quickly be made. In this way reflection and understanding can become possible. Better data may become available later, but it is not data that solve the problem, but the ideas arising from it. Even a small amount of information from fluctuations about to disappear will help to provide a starting point for future occasions.

13.2.1   Initial considerations

The first steps are to consider the problem along with the plant staff, and to determine the following.

(a) The nature of the problem; decide whether there has been a steady fall in yield, or whether periodic fluctuations are occurring.

(b) Make sure the problem is not due to infection.

As a first step it is advisable to visit the plant and obtain an understanding of the procedures used, and to identify any recent changes, both in working methods or in batch assessment. Collect any relevant analytical data, and also details of work that led to the adoption of the process under study. Results should be listed, so as to observe when the effects were first noticed, as this may be associated with a change in practice. For this, a control chart, as described later, can be very helpful.

New data on current batches should be obtained, and data on respiration are useful, as the batches may no longer be working within the oxygen-transfer capacity of the fermenters. It is important to be satisfied that the process is being operated correctly. Plant workers are usually very careful about this, but an investigator needs to be satisfied if only for the sake of his own mental clarity.

13.2.2   Information from different sources

The main sources of information are likely to be periodical plant data reports, together with information provided by the plant staff, from day-to-day records. There may also be relevant research information. Information from plant workers at all levels is usually of great importance, and this will consist of measurements and general observations. This will bring out the assumptions made about the process, and how the batch should look throughout its progress. The set of data items collected may not be the same as in the laboratory (cf. Fig. 12.1). Changes in pH are often given much attention, as they mark key events in the development of the batch. The plant workers' views on the successive changes that occur during batches are often very relevant, and they often have strong views about them. One expert has commented that folklore should also be collected, as this is a way of recording real events seen from another angle. The visiting researcher must remember that the solution is likely to arise from the plant team, since they are closest to the subject. These comments from plant staff should be carefully compared with laboratory experience.

The researcher should also be a source of ideas. Before the visit, attempts should be made to rationalise the position, using all the data available, and methods of diagnosis should also be prepared. These efforts may be unsuccessful, but they can produce a useful operating framework, capable of quick modification.

13.2.3   Causes of loss of productivity

The following are possible causes of reduced production.
(a) Rundown of the producer organism.
(b) A change in quality in one of the ingredients in the medium.
(c) A weakness in the metabolic system, triggered by a temporary occurrence during the batch or in the pre-production stages.
(d) An alteration in the process, made without realising it might upset production.
(e) Inaccurate instrumentation; for example, a thermometer.
(f) A change in the plant, which might have an unexpected effect.
(g) Infection: this possibility must be eliminated.

The main indicator of inefficiency is the reduction in antibiotic yield, but a detailed study of the pattern of growth and metabolism is likely to provide clues to the cause of the trouble, and this can be used to forecast the result of the fermentation.

Of these possibilities, (a) and (b) can be checked by using alternative culture and ingredients in fermentation trials. The culture can be plated and checked for variation. Regarding the ingredients, natural products are seasonal and can be obtained from different parts of the world at different times of the year. They can therefore vary in quality. It is known that some strains are sensitive to the triggering described in (c). Sensitivity may have appeared in the laboratory.

The variations described in (d), (e), and (f) should be checked, but this is often far from easy to do. Changes may arise from convenience or from a new policy, with the assumption that they will make no difference. In some plants, temperature control may be difficult in warm weather, while temporary stoppages of stirring or aeration sometimes occur during maintenance work or from a power failure.

The size and complexity of the plant make it difficult to check all possible variations in the process, while process operations are not always easy to follow, especially as an 8-day production batch may extend over 16 days if the pre-production stages are included, and many groups of workers are likely to be involved. It is necessary to visualise all the practical operations involved and to decide their importance in the resulting batch so that all the critical steps can be checked.

When the investigation is over, it is often difficult to be certain as to the cause of the problem. Quite often normal working seems to return spontaneously. It is, however, usually possible to identify the cause quite well, though there is usually a feeling that the trouble, having been driven away, is only too ready to come back again.

13.2.4   Big and little factors in efficiency

The discussion in the previous section dealing with the causes of reduced production brings out a more general subject which will be mentioned briefly. In the consideration of antibiotic fermentations and the way they work, there is a tendency to think in terms of major factors, such as the cells' physiological and biochemical behaviour, material flows, oxygen transfer, and the relation between growth and production. These are the 'big' factors in productivity, which naturally attract the academic side of our thinking.

It has to be realised, though, that in the works it is often the little factors that emerge as dominant. These include matters like temperature control, detailed operation of the seed and pre-production cultures, steady conditions during the production fermentation, and a host of other details that are essential to success. In laboratory work these tend to be overlooked because the working area is smaller and staff supervision is greater. Additionally, if a laboratory batch fails, it can usually be discarded and repeated, something impossible in the plant. Thus the effect of the 'little' factors is missed unless the occasion is striking. In the middle of a Ph.D. programme, when the production of spores in shaken flasks was essential to start the research fermentations, the spore flask cultures remained white instead of turning dark green. The situation was saved by finding an alternative master culture at the back of the refrigerator. Historically the event never occurred. The importance of a little factor had become apparent. Such little factors also often appear when teaching in the laboratory. Specimen plates for the students to examine are all 'atypical' because they were put in the wrong incubator, or there was a mistake in the medium. The basic importance of these little factors should never be forgotten in process development investigations.

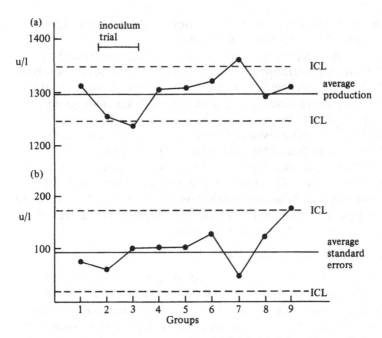

Fig. 13.2. Control chart for a series of antibiotic batches. The graphs show (a) averaged production points for groups of four batches with (b) their standard errors points. Also shown are the population average lines and the inner control limits (ICL, $P = 0.025$) for both production and standard error. Productivity is expressed in arbitrary units/litre (u/l).

13.2.5   Analysis of data by control chart

When studying the serial production of items, which vary to some extent, it is convenient to use a control chart. This technique, too long to describe here in detail, will be found in the literature, e.g. Davies (1967). In this method, the averages of small groups of products are plotted in series, along with their standard errors. Inner and outer control limits are also plotted, based on the variation of the whole population. For example, the inner control limits (ICL) give the likely chance variation arising from the observed standard error (SE) assuming a probability coefficient (P) of 0.025. If the group average points fall within these limits, the variation is probably due to chance; if they fall outside, it is likely that a true source of variation is present.

   In the case of an antibiotic, a marked fall in plant productivity was observed, and the question arose as to whether it was a real effect and whether a cause could be attributed to it. In this case, batch results over several months were divided into groups of four, and the control chart shown in Fig. 13.2 was prepared, using the method of Davies (1967). This shows the averages for production and for the standard errors, along with the inner control limits. The error average seems high, compared with productivity, since a certain amount was deducted from the production data. The averaging procedure, used in the control chart, has the advantage of smoothing the graphs, which can become highly complex if individual batch results are plotted.

In the example, the groups 2 and 3 showed a significant fall in productivity compared with the others, the error range being close to average. The other groups seemed normal except for 7 and 9. The effects observed with these were due to individual aberrant batches, such as occur occasionally. As to the low productivity in groups 2 and 3, it was found on enquiry that a change had been made in the preparation of the seed cultures. This was convenient and seemed harmless, but it had an unfortunate effect.

The control chart thus gives a useful overview. It is helpful in examining a series of results and also in picking out individual effects of special interest. The value of the accompanying chart of the standard error is also useful, as it detects periods when the process goes out of control, as shown by the values reaching or exceeding the control limits.

In this case, as with others, the problem was essentially detective work. Sherlock Holmes used to say that when all other possibilities had been eliminated, what remained must be the explanation of what took place. Although in trouble-shooting it is often not possible to identify every possibility, the saying is still a useful starting point for the investigator.

13.3   Major fluctuations in the level of antibiotic production

The occurrence of large fluctuations in yield can be a serious problem in plant work. Such behaviour is also not unfamiliar in teaching practical microbiology, and it is overcome by the skill of technicians in the choice of strains and growth conditions, resulting in smooth presentations in the laboratory. This type of behaviour has been referred to by Hockenhull & McKenzie (1968), who refer to batches that do not get off on the right foot, and presented in more detail by Dr S. W. Carleysmith (1985, unpublished) in the course of a lecture on plant operations, and it is probably quite well known to industrial workers. It is possible that it relates to the regulatory system in the high-yielding mutants used, in which deleterious gene arrangements have accumulated along with high-yielding ones, thus producing excessive sensitivity to culture conditions (Rowlands & Normansell, 1983).

In manufacture, these fluctuations present a practical problem. Signs of deviation from normal may become apparent to the shift supervisor, but his successor may not agree, and there may be some confusion. If a serious fluctuation can be detected, it may be possible to take action, such

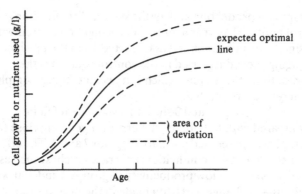

Fig. 13.3. Growth and nutrient use in deviant batches.

as continuing the batch for a shortened span, or by killing the organism by heating to 60 °C and re-inoculating, or by adding glucose to return the cells to a vegetative state, giving them a chance to return to a more productive condition. In some cases the fluctuation may alter the pH, and adjustment can be made. Obviously this decision must be taken early, and a new batch programme arranged.

Batch variations of this kind can occur in the laboratory as well as in the plant. Conditions are simpler in the laboratory since costs are relatively low and a re-start is the usual response. A study of some of these deviant batches might be useful in providing clues to the situation under plant conditions.

13.3.1   Metabolic aspects of the fluctuations

The sketch in Fig. 13.3 provides a basis for the consideration of deviant batches. A line is shown, representing the expected growth curve for optimal production. A corresponding line could also represent the consumption of a particular nutrient, which would also have an optimal shape, but the curves for growth and consumption would probably differ. Instead of a single line, therefore, a real batch would show a family of curves, each corresponding to a particular factor. The curve for antibiotic production, related to these other lines, could also vary. In Fig. 13.3 the dashed lines indicate that there is an area over which these lines can vary, as batches deviate from normal.

The cause of these disturbances from the optimal pattern could lie in small changes in conditions or variations in natural products in the medium. These would alter the rates of breakdown and utilisation, possibly affecting the pH and requiring correction by addition of acid or alkali. More fundamentally, they could arise from the microbial culture itself, expressed particularly in variations in its metabolism and internal regulation.

As a result of these changes, the nature of the fermentation can alter altogether and can no longer be regarded as being in the original mould. The variations from normal are no longer around a basic mean but belong to a different order of society. If a mental image has been formed on some sort of basis as that in Fig. 4.1, then all the relations between the components have become changed. The practical problem is the detection of these changes, so that allowance can be made in the batch process to deal with them. The approaches described arise from experience, and from a discussion of the subject in a lecture by Dr S. W. Carleysmith (1985, unpublished).

While Fig. 13.3 has stressed the growth curve, it is probable that growth curves do not vary as much as might be expected during the early stages of aberrant batches, so that it would be better to base the analysis of the position on the curves for other factors, especially those closely linked to antibiotic biosynthesis.

It will be recognised that the discussion of the problem of variations in performance involves several aspects: whether variations can be detected at an early stage; what methods could be used to detect them; and how the position could be established from them. The discussion of these points is necessarily speculative, but it introduces an interesting area of industrial microbiology and biochemistry.

13.3.2   Can variations be observed early, so that action can be taken?

A few examples are available that suggest that this possibility exists. In these, the variations occurred when using constant fermentation conditions. Changes in culture patterns, with different working conditions, are described in Chapters 5 and 6.

By direct observation
When the inoculum is added to a production culture, it is possible to judge at quite an early stage whether the yield is likely to be high or low. This may be based on the appearance of the culture and changes such as the appearance of a tinge of colour and an odour, indicating the onset of secondary metabolism at the correct time. Experienced workers are skilled at making this judgement, but its reliability is not always certain. Delayed appearance of colour may indicate that the fermentation is behind and will return to normal after a few hours. Different workers also may make their judgement on the basis of different features, and colour shades may be distinguished in different ways, for example pink or yellow, against reddish or brownish.

Another method of evaluation is the use of microscopic examination. Some workers make an extreme use of this method, which is certainly of some value. This again has the difficulty of subjectivity, while the changes observed may be difficult to describe and are basically complex.

Table 13.2. *Enzyme concentrations in inoculum, and yields in griseofulvin batches*

Batch quality	high yield	low yield
Number of batches	1	4
Enzyme		
G6PDH (mU/mg cells)	9.4	20.3
ICDH (mU/mg cells)	8.9	4.2
Ratio	1:1	4.8:1

Although these direct methods have the risk of subjectivity, they have the advantage of immediacy and rapidity. With some degree of standardisation they are bound to be used as a first characterisation step.

By enzyme measurements
In Chapter 4.4, the variation of enzyme concentrations in the mycelium of inoculum cultures was shown to be related to productivity. Smith & Calam (1980) have described the variations of inocula giving rise to high- and low-yielding griseofulvin batches, the latter giving about 60% of normal. Values in the inoculum cultures are shown in Table 13.2. The results show a clear difference.

The production batches also showed differences in enzyme contents, as previously described with penicillin experiments (Chapter 4.4) when different inocula were used. Results are given in Table 13.3. The later and broader peak in enzyme concentrations is well marked in the lower-yielding batches, suggesting a different introduction to the production phase, which began at 120 h. The growth curves were very similar in both low- and high-yielding batches.

Another example noted by Al-Jawadi (1984) related to shaken cultures producing oxytetracycline, giving high and low yields for no apparent reason. In the high-yielding fermentations, the level of acetyl-CoA carboxylase was twice as high at 24 h, before production started, as with low yielders.

The measurement of enzyme concentrations is not difficult, takes only a short time, and is suitable for routine use. The evidence from these experiments suggests this approach could be of considerable utility, but the amount of evidence available is scattered and needs further investigation.

By measurement of K_{La}
In describing the measurement of the oxygen transfer coefficient K_{La} by an indirect dynamic method (Bandyopadhyay, Humphrey & Taguchi, 1967), it was implied that the method could be used in scale-up work, and it has also been suggested the K_{La} could be used to indicate the structure of a mycelial culture, its structure being related to the degree of inhibition of gas transfer.

Table 13.3. *Enzyme levels in griseofulvin production batches*

Age of batch (h)	High yield			low yield		
	Enzyme conc. (mU/mg dry cells)			Enzyme conc. (mU/mg dry cells)		
	ICDH	G6PDH	cells (g/l)	ICDH	G6PDH	cells (g/l)
25	19	22	10	13	18	9
50	19	29	22	21	27	24
75	13	24	29.5	23	33	34
100	9	15	33	19	31	36.5
125	7	9	34	10	21	35

Some data recorded by Ismail (1977) were suitable for testing this possibility; it was based on a series of penicillin fermentations carried out in laboratory fermenters. These include batches giving normal and sub-normal yields. The latter occurred for no apparent reason and resembled the deviant batches referred to here. The results obtained are shown in Table 13.4, which shows cell growth, carbon dioxide production (used as an index of oxygen uptake), and the concentration of dissolved oxygen, along with penicillin production. Although there was some variation among the results, the averages give a good indication of the effects observed. With synthetic and with corn-steep media, the value of K_{La} at 24 h was a good indicator of the future level of productivity, though otherwise the batches were very similar. There was no distinction with the peanut medium, probably because there was a high level of dissolved matter at first (cf. Batch 36, described in Chapter 8.2.3. and Fig. 8.2).

The results suggest that the oxygen transfer coefficient appears to have a useful potential in identifying culture quality, though measurement in plant batches might be difficult due to the fragility of the oxygen electrodes. For experimental purposes it might be possible to transfer a large sample of culture to a laboratory fermenter, where the necessary measurements could be made without difficulty.

Taking the results together, there is a good indication that batch quality can be detected at an early age by considering fungal state (K_{La}) or by biochemical quality (enzyme activity) or by observation. In a given fermentation, the details of these matters would require detailed investigation.

13.3.3   The assessment of culture quality

Since it may be necessary to monitor batches so that variations from the normal can be detected, a brief account of possible approaches to the problem will be attempted. This is perhaps risky, because each type of

Table 13.4. *Variations of* K_{La} *with high- and low-yielding batches*

Media and parameters	No. of batches averaged	Low yield (72 h)	High yield (72 h)
Synthetic medium	3		
Penicillin (u/ml)		2750	5066
CO_2 (%) 24 h		1.41	1.07
K_{La}			
24 h		419	263
36 h		521	249
Dry cells (g/l at 48 h)		20.8	26.5
Corn-steep medium	3–4		
Penicillin (u/ml)		4570	6263
CO_2 (%) 24 h		1.11	1.01
K_{La}			
24 h		267	155
36 h		453	156
Dry cells (g/l at 48 h)		39.0	37.8
Peanut medium	2		
Penicillin (u/ml)		4300	6550
CO_2 (%)		0.90	1.04
K_{La}			
24 h		127	132
36 h		221	165
Dry matter (g/l at 48 h)		49.7	45.5

Trials with 5-l fermenters, aerated at 1 v/v/m, and with different types of media (averaged data; K_{La} per hour).

antibiotic fermentation is different, but some generalisation is possible.

A list of tests that might be used is given in Table 13.5, which is divided into three sections.

The first section gives methods for estimating growth in terms of growth and appearance. These subjects have already been discussed above.

The second section gives some measurements that can be related to growth and the type of culture produced. The first three, related to respiration, have already been discussed, while viscosity follows in this area of work. Requirement for alkali for pH control in another measure, directly related to growth and metabolism. Heat evolution is a possibility that has been referred to in the literature. Of the other two, the use of ATP to estimate cell concentrations is described in the literature, and certain firms, for example New Brunswick and LKB, provide equipment and reagents for quick, routine tests. The use of the methylene-blue reduction test and the concentration of amino-pimelic acid to estimate

Table 13.5. *Methods for culture assessment*

---

(1) Methods for direct observation of growth
Direct measurement of cell concentration, by filtration, drying, and weighing
[a] Packed cell volume
[a] Degree of settling on standing
[a] Appearance of culture, pelleting, etc. in dish
[a] Colour, appearance, and odour of sample

(2) Measurements related to growth
Respiration: oxygen uptake, CO_2 output, dissolved oxygen, RQ
[a] Spot readings of carbon dioxide
K_{La} or dynamic K_{La}
[a] Viscosity (by Brookfield viscometer)
Alkali requirement for pH control
Heat evolution from use of cooling water
[a] Concentration of ATP in cells
[a] Methylene-blue reduction, and content of diaminopimelic acid

(3) Metabolic effects
[a] pH, or change in pH over a given time
[a] Disappearance or concentration of sugar, amino acids, ammonia, and other substances
Appearance of antibiotic
Background chromatograms (HPLC) for organic substances, recognised by fluorescence or UV absorption, or for residual inorganic substances, e.g. phosphate, Mg, K, etc.
Concentration in cells of enzymes such as diastase and protease, or of specialised enzymes ICDH, G6PDH, MDH
Behaviour of filtered cells in buffer, measured by using respirometer or by shaking in buffer with selected nutrients and measuring products after a few hours

---

[a] *Relatively quick and simple.*

growth are described by Bosnjak, Topolovec & Vrana (1978) in a paper on the control of the erythromycin fermentation.

In the third section, a number of more-complex possibilities are listed. These are based on studies of the state and changes in the metabolism of the cells during the fermentation. These centre around the removal of nutrients from the medium, which usually occurs in a stepwise manner, and the appearance of intermediates for biosynthesis and the product itself. It also suggests that the changes in concentration of inorganic elements can usefully be followed. The possibilities of using enzyme concentrations as diagnostics has already been discussed. Tests of samples transferred to special media in shaken flasks is also a possible approach.

Some of these tests imply a complicated analytical system. In these times such systems are not uncommon, for example in the production of fermented foods and beverages, using gas–liquid chromatography (GLC) or HPLC to give patterns of components important to the system. Mathers *et al.* (1986) have used a computer-HPLC system to monitor a fermentation. Nolan (1986) has described a test system for new antibiotics, based on their action on a number of enzymes. The enzyme activities were measured semi-automatically and recorded by a computer, which compared the results, for novelty, against a stored data list.

While the organisation and introduction of such systems to a fermentation plant control room would require a great deal of research and effort, it would seem likely that methods of this kind may well be in use, to a partial or full extent, to provide guidance to controllers and plant operators.

In this connection, it may be mentioned that in dyestuffs manufacture, circular paper chromatograms have been used for over 50 years to follow the production of the colour and disappearance of intermediates during the chemical conversion. For this a large filter paper is held between two glass plates, the upper plate having a hole in the centre, through which drops of the reaction mixture are added. The pattern of rings that develops provides the necessary information within a few minutes. In cement production, the mixture of chalk, clay, and other substances must give the exact balance of the elements involved. In a modern plant, the controller has an automatic X-ray analyser linked to a computer to analyse the raw materials, the results being presented in 100 sec. A second computer is programmed to calculate the correct mixture. Thus the types of analyses required are far from impractical.

13.3.4   Diagnosis of batch condition

Tests with laboratory and plant batches would be needed to provide the correct linkages between the measurements of the various components and the state of the batch (either normal, or in some way abnormal). These investigations would lead to a computer identification programme, possibly based on an expert system, to identify the state of the batch and to prescribe the necessary action, such as that described in Chapter 11.3.6.

Such a diagnostic system would probably involve several stages, an initial one to decide whether the position was normal or whether attention was needed, followed by further testing to clarify the position. One of the advantages here of computerised reading of the test results is the possibility of rapid transfer of the information to the diagnostic programme, so as to give a quick and reliable result without the need for the transfer of written information.

The subjects dealt with in this chapter are of great importance in plant operations and have a considerable impact on development work. Although the discussion has had to be speculative and limited in scope, it is offered as an illustration of the sorts of problems that have to be tackled in practice, and the methods of thinking and working that have to be developed. It is therefore hoped that it has not been without value.

Postscript

Reviewing the field of antibiotic process development, it can be seen to be a mixture of chance, biochemical and physiological understanding, and the adaptation of a biological process to a physical framework defined by the fermentation equipment.

In wild strains, antibiotic production forms part of the system of differentiation that lies behind the cycle of growth and reproduction; it is usually associated with the end of vegetative growth and the onset of sporulation. Such a rigid system is unsuited to development, and the initial stages of mutation and selection have the effect of loosening this linkage so that antibiotic production starts to extend over a longer period of growth. Thus, at this stage, production often appears to be growth linked and to be associated with a particular phase of growth that must be extended as long as possible. Later on in development, growth and production become relatively independent, and production can be maintained over a long period, giving very high production levels. This often requires that the cells be grown in a particular form of pellets, enabling the productive phase to be held for many days.

There are two obvious limitations to high levels of production, first the supply of oxygen for energy production (and possibly for the maintenance of a favourable aerobic balance in the cells), second the inhibitory effect of the antibiotic and of other products in the fermentation. With wild strains, many substances are inhibitory, such as phosphate, but many of these effects are lost in mutation. Glucose, however, usually remains inhibitory to antibiotic production.

In fermentations giving maximum production, a complex balance has to be maintained during the fermentation. This balance is usually obtained by the use of complex media and a system of feeding, often with more than one component.

The metabolism of producer strains is very sensitive to culture conditions, and the selection of very-high-yielding strains becomes difficult on this account. It is not uncommon for a new strain to work well in the laboratory but fail in the plant because of its inability to accommodate itself to the changed conditions. The problems that lie in this field are difficult to solve and account for the fact that very extensive pilot-plant work is needed for success. Development work in the main plant is not difficult microbiologically, but the nature of the plant and the

200

complexity of the work require a new approach in the development field.

Underlying the gradual development of new strains and processes is the problem of the microorganism itself. The change from a wild strain to a very-high-yielding industrial strain involves a very large number of mutations and, in addition, very many choices as the best isolates are selected at each step on the way. Thus, in the best isolates, it is possible to build up not only advantageous mutations that give high yields, but also disadvantageous mutations that build up trouble as development continues. This leads to unstable fermentation systems, which are difficult to keep in balance and require further efforts at plant level to ensure steady production. These disadvantageous mutations also present a difficulty to selection workers, whose task is doubled in trying to make the best of both aspects of this subject.

So far, direct gene insertion has not made much impact on the scene, mainly because of the complexity of the antibiotic production process, and the lack of information on the exact genes that need manipulation. The possibility of gene insertion in connection with antibiotic production has been abundantly demonstrated, and most industrial firms are giving the work prominence. There are likely to be extensive developments over the next few years as the keys are found to a scientifically based approach to the situation.

Process development might be expected to be based on a scientific understanding of the fermentation mechanisms. Unfortunately the subject remains an observational science. On the other hand, a biochemical and physiological approach provides an invaluable background for thought and prediction and experimental planning. In some cases it has led to the discovery of precursors and inhibitors and provided ways to directly improve production. It is a field of the greatest interest, especially because it is linked with such a wide field of research. It is unfortunate that at present most of the information available arises from wild strains or low-yielding mutants. The higher the industrial firms are able to lift a corner of the curtain and give a better view of the way high-yielding strains actually behave, the better it will be for the science of industrial microbiology.

At the moment, as a rule, we have to consider each antibiotic as a member of a small group of related substances. Each group has its own behaviour patterns and theory, different from the other groups. Development remains a matter of imagination and the observation of chances, being based on observed and quantitative data. It is not possible to devise a universal development programme that covers every kind of antibiotic fermentation.

Bibliography

Burnett, J. H. & Trinci, A. J. P. (eds) (1979). *Fungal Walls and Hyphal Growth.* Cambridge University Press.

* Demain, A. L. & Solomon, N. A. (eds) (1986). *Manual of Industrial Microbiology and Biotechnology.* Washington, DC: American Society for Microbiology.

Goodfellow, M., Mordanski, M. & Williams, S. T. (eds) (1984). *Biology of Actinomycetes.* London: Academic Press.

Krumphangl, V., Sikyta, B. & Vaněk, Z. (eds) (1982). *Overproduction of Microbial Products.* London: Academic Press.

Nisbet, L. J. & Winstanley, D. J. (eds) (1983). *Bioactive Microbial Products 2, Development and Production.* London: Academic Press.

Old, R. W. & Primrose, S. B. (1981). *Principles of Gene Manipulation.* Oxford: Blackwell.

Riviere, J. (1977). *Industrial Applications of Microbiology,* transl. and ed. M. O. Moss & J. E. Smith. London: Surrey University Press.

Saunders, V. A. & Saunders, J. (1986). *Microbial Genetics Applied to Biotechnology.* London: Croome Hill.

Vandamme, E. J. (ed.) (1984). *Biotechnology of Industrial Antibiotics.* New York: Marcel Dekker.

* Vaněk, Z. & Hošťálek, Z. (eds) (1968). *Overproduction of Microbial Metabolites.* Boston, Mass.; Butterworth.

* These two recent books will be found to expand and fill out many areas of the present book.

References

Al-Jawadi, M. (1984). 'Biochemical and Morphological Changes in *Streptomyces rimosus* on Mutation to Higher Yields of Oxytetracycline'. Ph.D. Thesis, CNAA, London.

Al-Jawadi, M. & Calam, C. T. (1987). Physiology of a wild strain and high yielding mutants of *S. rimosus*, producing oxytetracycline. *Folia Microbiologica*, **32**, in press.

Al-Jawadi, M., Wellington, E. M. H. & Calam, C. T. (1985). Identification of some streptomycetes producing oxytetracycline. *Journal of General Microbiology*, **131**, 2241–4.

Auden J., Gruner, J., Knüsel, F. & Nüesch, J. (1967). Some statistical methods in nutrient medium optimisation. *Pathology and Microbiology*, **30**, 858–66.

Auerbach, C. (1976). *Mutation Research: Problems, Results and Perspectives.* London: Chapman & Hall.

Aytoun, R. S. & McWilliam, R. W. (1957). Improvements in the production of mutants of the genus *Penicillium*. British Patent 788,118.

Ball, C. (1983). Protoplast fusion in commercially important microorganisms. In *Bioactive Microbial Products 2, Development and Production*, ed. L. J. Nisbet & D. J. Winstanley, pp. 19–31. London: Academic Press.

Ball, C. & McGonagle, M. P. (1978). Development and evaluation of a potency index screen for detection of mutants of *Penicillium chrysogenum* having increased yield. *Journal of Applied Bacteriology*, **45**, 67–74.

Baltz, R. H. (1978). Genetic recombination in *Streptomyces fradiae* by protoplast fusion and cell regeneration. *Journal of General Microbiology*, **107**, 93–102.

Bandyopadhyay, B., Humphrey, A. E. & Taguchi, H. (1967). Dynamic method for K_{La}. *Biotechnology and Bioengineering*, **9**, 523–44.

Beecham Group Ltd (1968). Production of 6-amino-penicillanic acid. British Patent 1,118,566.

Bosnjak, M., Topolovec, V. & Vrana, M. (1978). Growth kinetics of *Streptomyces erythreus* during erythromycin biosynthesis. *Journal of Applied Chemistry and Biotechnology*, **28**, 791–8.

Box, G. E. P. & Wilson, K. B. (1951). On the experimental attainment of optimum conditions. *Journal of the Royal Statistical Society* B, **13**, 1.

Branch, J. (1986). Interacting with computers – expert systems. *Chemistry & Industry*, (1986), 321–4.

Bu'Lock, J. D., Comberbach, M. C., Ghomnich, C. & Williams, P. W. (1984). *Chemistry & Industry*, (1984), 432–4.

Bu'Lock, J. D., Detroy, R. W., Hošťálek, Z. & Munim-Al-Shakarchi, A. (1974). Regulation of secondary biosynthesis in *Gibberella fujikuroi*. *Transactions of the British Mycological Society*, **62**, 377–89.

Calam, C. T. (1964). The selection, improvement and preservation of microorganisms. *Progress in Industrial Microbiology*, **5**, 1–53.

Calam, C. T. (1969). The evaluation of mycelial growth. In *Methods in Microbiology*, vol. 1, ed. J. R. Norris & D. W. Ribbons, pp. 567–91. London: Academic Press.

Calam, C. T. (1970). Improvement of microorganisms by mutation, hybridisation and selection. In *Methods in Microbiology*, vol. 3A, ed. J. R. Norris & D. W. Ribbons, pp. 435–59. London: Academic Press.

Calam, C. T. (1982). Factors governing the production of penicillin by *Penicillium chrysogenum*. In *Overproduction of Microbial Products*, ed. V. Krumphanzl, B. Sikyta & Vaněk, Z., pp. 89–95. London: Academic Press.

Calam, C. T. (1986). Shake flask fermentations. In *Industrial Microbiology and Biotechnology*, ed. A. L. Demain & N. A. Solomon, pp. 59–65, Washington, DC: American Society for Microbiology.

Calam, C. T., Daglish, L. B. & Gaitskell, W. S. (1973). Hybridisation experiments with *Penicillium patulum* and *Fusarium moniliforme*. In *Genetics of Industrial Microorganisms*, vol. 2, ed. Z. Vaněk, Z. Hošťálek, & J. Cudlin, pp. 265–82. Prague: Academia.

Calam, C. T., Daglish, L. B. & McCann, E. P. (1976). Penicillin: tactics in strain improvement. In *Second International Symposium on the Genetics of Industrial Microorganisms*, ed. K. D. Macdonald, pp. 273–87. London: Academic Press.

Calam, C. T., Driver, N. & Bowers, R. H. (1951). Studies in the production of penicillin, respiration and growth of *Penicillium chrysogenum* in submerged culture, in relation to oxygen transfer. *Journal of Applied Chemistry*, 1, 209–16.

Calam, C. T., Ellis, S. H. & McCann, M. J. (1971). Mathematical models and a simulation of the grizeofulvin fermentation. *Journal of Applied Chemistry and Biotechnology*, 21, 181–9.

Calam, C. T. & Ismail, B.A.-K. (1980). Investigation of factors in the optimisation of penicillin production. *Journal of Chemical Technology and Biotechnology*, 30, 249–62.

Calam, C. T. & Russell, D. W. (1973). Microbial aspects of fermentation development. *Journal of applied Chemistry and Biotechnology*, 23, 255–37.

Calam, C. T. & Smith, G. M. (1981). Regulation of the biochemistry and morphology of *Penicillium chrysogenum*. *FEMS Microbiology Letters*, 10, 231–4.

Carter, B. L. A. & Bull, A. T. (1969). Studies of fungal growth and intermediary carbon metabolism under steady and non-steady conditions. *Biotechnology and Bioengineering*, 11, 785–804.

Chang, R. S. L., Lotti, V. J., Monaghan, R. L., Birnbaum, J., Stapley, E. O., Goertz, M. A., Albers-Schönberg, G., Patchett, A. A., Liersch, J. M., Hensens, O. D. & Springer, J. P. (1985). A potent non-peptide cholecystokinin antagonist selective for peripheral tissues isolated from *Aspergillus alliaceus*. *Science*, 230, 177–9.

Chater, K. F. & Merrick, M. J. (1976) Approaches to the study of differentiation in *Streptomyces coelicolor* A3(2). In *Second International Symposium on the Genetics of Industrial Microorganisms*, ed. K. D. Macdonald, pp. 583–94. London: Academic Press.

Collins, J. F. (1976). Gene amplification in bacterial systems. In *second International Symposium on the Genetics of Industrial Microorganisms*, ed. K. D. Macdonald, pp. 41–58. London: Academic Press.

Conn, E. E. & Stumpf, P. K. (1976). *Outline of Biochemistry*, 4th ed. New York: John Wiley.

Constantinides, A., Spencer, J. & Gaden, E. L., Jr (1970). Development of mathematical models of batch penicillin fermentation. *Biotechnology and Bioengineering*, **12**, 803–30.

Davies, O. L. (1964). Screening for improved mutants in antibiotic research. *Biometrics*, **20**, 576–91.

Davies, O. L. (ed.) (1967). *The Design and Analysis of Industrial Experiments*, 2nd edn. London: Oliver & Boyd.

Demain, A. L. (1957). Inhibition of penicillin formation by lysine. *Archives of Biochemistry and Biophysics*, **67**, 244–5.

Demain, A. L. (1982). Catabolite regulation in industrial microbiology. In *Overproduction of Microbial Products*, ed. B. Krumphanzl, B. Sikyta & Z. Vaněk, pp. 3–20. London: Academic Press.

Demain, A. L. (1983). Foreword. In *Secondary Metabolism and Differentiation*, ed. J. W. Bennett & A. Ciegler, p. v. New York: Marcel Dekker.

Demain, A. L. & Solomon, N. A. (eds) (1986). *Manual of Industrial Microbiology and Technology*. Washington, DC: American Society for Microbiology.

Drew, S. W. & Demain, A. L. (1975). Stimulation of cephalosporin production by methionine peptides in a mutant blocked in reverse transsulfuration. *Journal of Antibiotics*, **28**, 889–95.

Duckworth, R. B. & Harris, G. C. M. (1949). The morphology of *Penicillium chrysogenum* in submerged fermentations. *Transactions of the British Mycological Society*, **32**, 224–35.

Elander, R. P. (1982). Traditional *versus* current approaches to genetic improvement of microbial strains. In *Overproduction of Microbial Products*, ed. V. Krumphanzl, B. Sikyta & Z. Vaněk, pp. 353–70. London: Academic Press.

Frank, M. C., Calam, C. T. & Gregory, P. H. (1948). The production of spores by *Penicillium notatum*. *Journal of General Microbiology*, **2**, 70–9.

Gaden, E. L., Jr (1959). Fermentation process kinetics. *Journal of Biochemical and Microbial Technology*, **1**, 413–29.

Ghisalba, O., Traxler, P. & Nüesch, J. (1978). Early intermediates in the biosynthesis of ansamycins. I. Isolation and identification of protorifamycin. *Journal of Antibiotics*, **31**, 1124–31.

Gräfe, U., Reinhardt, G., Krebs, D., Eritt, I. & Fleck, W. F. (1984). Pleiotropic effects of a butyrolactone-type auto-regulator on mutants of *Streptomyces griseus* blocked in cytodifferentiation. *Journal of General Microbiology*, **130**, 1237–45.

Gray, P. P. & Bhuwapathanapun, S. (1980). Production of the macrolide antibiotic tylosin in batch and chemostat cultures. *Biotechnology and Bioengineering*, **22**, 1785–1804.

Hara, O., Horinouchi, S. & Uozumi, T. (1983). Genetic analysis of A-factor synthesis in *Streptomyces coelicolor* A3(2) and *Streptomyces griseus*. *Journal of General Microbiology*, **129**, 2939–44.

Harold, R. L. H. & Harold, F. M. (1986). Ionophores and cytochlasins modulate branching in *Achlya bisexualis*. *Journal of General Microbiology*, **132**, 312–19.

Hersbach, G. J. M., Van der Beek, C. P. & Van dijck, P. W. M. (1984). The penicillins: properties, biosynthesis and fermentation. In *Biotechnology of Industrial Antibiotics*, ed. E. J. Vandamme, pp. 45–140. New York: Marcel Dekker.

206   References

Heyes, W. F. (1978). The biosynthesis and commercial production of neomycin – a review. *Process Biochemistry*, **13** (No. 12), 10–20.

Hockenhull, D. J. D. (1961). Improvements relating to antibiotics. British Patent 868,958.

Hockenhull, D. J. D. & McKenzie, R. M. (1968). Preset nutrient feeds for penicillin fermentation on defined media. *Chemistry and Industry*, (1968), 607–10.

Hopwood, D.A. (1970). The isolation of mutants. In *Methods in Microbiology*, Vol. 3A, ed. J. R. Norris & D. W. Ribbons, pp. 363–433. London: Academic Press.

Hopwood, D. A. & Wright, H. M. (1976). Genetic studies on SCP1-prime strains of *Streptomyces coelicolor*. *Journal of General Microbiology*, **95**, 107–20.

Hopwood, D. A. & Wright, H. M. (1979). Factors affecting recombinant frequency in protoplast fusion is *Streptomyces coelicolor*. *Journal of General Microbiology*, **111**, 137–43.

Hopwood, D. A. & Wright, H. M. (1981). Protoplast fusion in streptomycetes: fusion involving ultra-violet irradiated protoplasts. *Journal of General Microbiology*, **126**, 21–7.

Hopwood, D. A., Wright, H. M., Bibb, M. J. & Cohen, S. N. (1977). Genetic recombination through protoplast fusion in streptomycetes. *Nature*, **268**, 171–4.

Hosler, P. & Johnson, M. J. (1953). Penicillin from chemically defined media. *Industrial and Engineering Chemistry*, **45**, 871–4.

Hoštálek, Z. (1964). Relationship between the carbohydrate metabolism of *Streptomyces aureofasciens* and the biosynthesis of chlortetracycline. I. The effect of interrupted aeration, inorganic phosphate and benzyl thiocyanate on chlortetracycline biosynthesis. *Folia microbiologica*, **9**, 78–87.

Hoštálek, Z. & Vaněk, Z. (1973). Molecular basis of polygenic inheritance in the biosynthesis of chlortetracycline. In *Genetics of Industrial Microorganisms*, vol. 2, ed. Z. Vaněk, Z. Hoštálek & J. Cudlin, pp. 353–71. Prague: Academia.

Huber, F. M. & Tietz, A. J. (1983). Defined medium strategies for the biosynthesis of Cephalosporin C. *Biotechnology Letters*, **5**, 385–90.

Imperial Chemical Industries Ltd (1975). Liquid circulation and gas contacting device. British Patent 1,417,486.

Ismail, B.A.-K. (1977). 'A Study of the Factors in the Optimisation of the Penicillin Fermentation'. Unpublished Ph.D. thesis, CNAA, London.

Johnson, M. J., Stefaniak, J. J., Gailey, F. B. & Olson, B. H. (1946). Penicillin production by a superior strain of mold. *Science*, **103**, 504–5.

Khoklov, A. S. (1982). Low molecular weight microbial bioregulators in secondary metabolism. In *Overproduction of Microbial Products*, ed. V. Krumphanzl, B. Sikyta & Z. Vaněk, pp. 97–109, London: Academic Press.

König, B., Schügerl, K. & Seewald, S. (1982). Strategies for penicillin fermentation in Tower-loop reactors. *Biotechnology and Bioengineering*, **24**, 259–80.

Küenzi, M. T. & Auden, J. A. L. (1983). Design and control of fermentation processes. In *Bioactive Microbial Products 2, Development and Production*, ed. L. J. Nisbet & D. J. Winstanley, pp. 91–116. London: Academic Press.

Lein, J. (1986). The Pan Labs strain improvement programme. In *Overproduction of Microbial Metabolites*, ed. Z. Vaněk & Z. Hoštálek, pp. 105–40. Boston, Mass.: Butterworth.

Lilly, M. D. (1983). Problems in process scale-up. In *Bioactive microbial products 2, Development and Production*, ed. L. J. Nisbet & D. J. Winstanley, pp. 79–89. London: Academic Press.

McCann, E. P. & Calam, C. T. (1972). The metabolism of *Penicillium chrysogenum* and the production of penicillin using a high-yielding strain, at different temperatures. *Journal of Applied Chemistry and Biotechnology*, **22**, 1201–8.

Mandelstam, J. (1969). Regulation of bacterial spore formation. In *Microbial Growth*, ed. P. M. Meadow & S. J. Pirt, pp. 377–401. Cambridge University Press.

Martin, J. F. & Demain, A. L. (1980). Control of antibiotic synthesis. *Microbiological Reviews*, **44**, 230–51.

Martin, J. F., Luengo, J. M., Revilla, G. & Villanueva, J. R. (1979). Biochemical genetics of the β-lactam antibiotic biosynthesis. *Genetics of Industrial Microorganisms*, ed. O.K. Sebek & A. I. Laskin, pp. 83–9. Washington, DC: American Society for Microbiology.

Mathers, J. J., Dinwoodie, R. C., Talarovich, M. & Mehnert, D. W. (1986). Computer linked HPLC system for feedback control of fermentation substrates. *Biotechnology Letters*, **8**, 311–14.

Miles Laboratories Inc. (1952). Production of citric acid by fermentation. British Patent 672,128.

Mou, D. G. & Cooney, C. L. (1983*a*). Growth monitoring and control through computer-aided on-line mass balancing in a fed-batch penicillin fermentation. *Biotechnology and Bioengineering*, **25**, 225–55.

Mou, D. G. & Cooney, C. L. (1983*b*). Growth monitoring in complex medium: a case study employing a fed-batch penicillin fermentation and computer-aided mass-balancing. *Biotechnology and Bioengineering*, **25**, 257–69.

Nelligan, I. & Calam, C. T. (1980). Experience in the computer control of yeast growth. *Biotechnology Letters*, **2**, 531–6.

Nelligan, I. & Calam, C. T. (1983). Optimal control of penicillin production, using a mini-computer. *Biotechnology Letters*, **5**, 561–6.

Nolan, R. D. (1986). Partly automated system for strain improvement and secondary metabolite detection. *In Overproduction of microbial metabolites*, ed. Z. Vaněk & Z. Hošťálek, pp. 215–30. Boston, Mass.: Butterworth.

Normansell, D. (1982). Strain improvement in antibiotic producing microorganisms. *Journal of Chemical Technology and Biotechnology*, **32**, 296–303.

Old, R. W. & Primrose, S. B. (1981). *Principles of gene manipulation*, 2nd ed. Oxford: Blackwell Science Publishers.

Owen, S. P. & Johnson, M. J. (1955). Effect of temperature on the production of penicillin by *Penicillium chrysogenum*. *Applied Microbiology*, **3**, 375–9.

Peberdy, J. F. (1979). Fungal protoplasts. Isolation reversion and fusion. *Annual Reviews of Microbiology*, **33**, 21–39.

Peberdy, J. F. & Gibson, R. K. (1971). Regeneration of *Aspergillus nidulans* protoplasts. *Journal of General Microbiology*, **69**, 325–30.

Pirt, S. J. & Righelato, R. C. (1967). Effect of growth rate on the synthesis of penicillin in *Penicillium chrysogenum* in batch and chemostat cultures. *Applied Microbiology*, **15**, 1284–90.

Pogell, B. M. (1979). Regulation of aerial mycelium formation in streptomycetes. In *Genetics of Industrial Microorganisms*, ed. O.K. Sebek & A. I. Laskin, pp. 218–24. Washington, DC: American Society for Microbiology.

208   *References*

Pontecorvo, G., Roper, J. A. & Forbes, E. (1953). Genetic recombination without sexual recombination. *Journal of General Microbiology*, **8**, 198–210.

Pridham, T. G. & Tresner, H. D. (1974). Streptomyces, Waksman & Henrici 1943. In *Bergey's Manual of Determinative Bacteriology*, 8th edn, ed. R. E. Buchanan & N. F. Gibbons, pp. 748–829. Baltimore: Williams & Wilkins.

Prosser, J. I. & Trinci, A. J. P. (1979). A model for hyphal growth and branching. *Journal for General Microbiology*, **111**, 153–64.

Queener, S. & Swartz, R. (1979). The penicillins: biosynthetic and semi-synthetic. In *Secondary Products of metabolism*, ed. A. H. Rose, pp. 35–122. London: Academic Press.

Rhodes, A., Boothroyd, B. & Somerfield, G. A. (1961). Biosynthesis of griseofulvin: methylated benzophenone. *Biochemical Journal*, **81**, 28–37.

Rhodes, A., Crosse, R., Primrose, F. & Fletcher, D. L. (1957). Improvements in or relating to the production of the antibiotic griseofulvin. British Patent 784,618.

Rhodes, P. M., Hunter, I. S., Friend, E. J. & Warren, M. (1984). Recombinant methods for oxytetracycline producer *Streptomyces rimosus*. *Biochemical Society Transactions*, **12**, 586–7.

Rhodes, P. M., Winskill, N., Friend, E. J. & Warren, M. (1981). Biochemical and genetic characteristics of *S. rimosus* mutants impaired in oxytetracycline. *Journal of General Microbiology*, **124**, 329–38.

Richtie, G. (1985). From discovery to commercial reality, some aspects of fermentation product development. *Chemistry & Industry*, (1985) 403–7.

Righelato, R. C., Trinci, A. P. J., Pirt, S. J. & Peat, A. (1968). The influence of maintenance energy and growth rate on the metabolic activity morphology and conidiation of *Penicillium chrysogenum*. *Journal of General Microbiology*, **50**, 399–412.

Robbers, J. E. & Floss, R. G. (1976). Induction by tryptophane of ergot alkaloid biosynthesis. In *Nova Acta Leopoldina*, Supplement No. 7, *Leopoldina Symposium: Secondary metabolism and co-evolution*, ed. M. Luckner, K. Mothes & L. Nover, pp. 243–69. Halle (Saale): Deutsche Akademie der Naturforscher Leopoldina.

Roberts, S. M. (1984). β-Lactams, past and present. *Chemistry and Industry* (1984), 162–6.

Ross, N. G. & Wilkin, G. D. (1966). Continuous microbiological processes involving filamentous microorganisms. British Patent 1,133,875.

Rowlands, R. T. & Normansell, I. D. (1983). Current strategies in industrial selection. In *Bioactive Microbial Products 2, Development and Production*, ed. L. J. Nisbet & D. J. Winstanley, pp. 1–18. London: Academic Press.

Ryu, D.D.Y. & Hospodka, J. (1980). Quantitative physiology of *Penicillium chrysogenum* in penicillin fermentations. *Biotechnology and Bioengineering*, **22**, 289–97.

Ryu, D. D. Y. & Humphrey, A. E. (1973). Examples of computer-aided fermentation systems. *Journal of Applied Chemistry & Biotechnology*, **23**, 283–95.

Senior, P. J. & Windass, J. (1980). The ICI single cell protein process. *Biotechnology Letters*, **2**, 205–10.

Sermonti, G. (1969). *Genetics of Antibiotic Producing Microorganisms*. London: Wiley Interscience.

Shu, P. (1961). Mathematical models for the product accumulation in microbiological processes. *Journal of Biochemical and Microbiological Technology and Engineering*, **3**, 95–100.

Shu, P. & Johnson, M. J. (1945). Citric acid production by submerged fermentation with *Aspergillus niger*. *Industrial and Engineering Chemistry*, **40**, 1202–5.

Simpson, I. N. & Caten, C. E. (1981). Selection for increased penicillin titre following hybridisation of divergent lines of *Aspergillus nidulans. Journal of General Microbiology*, **126**, 311–19.

Smith, G. M. & Calam, C. T. (1980). Variations in inocula and their influence on the productivity of antibiotic fermentations. *Biotechnology Letters*, **2**, 261–6.

Smith, J. E. & Galbraith, J. C. (1971). Biochemical and physiological aspects of differentiation in the fungi. *Advances in Microbial Physiology*, **5**, 45–62.

Society of Chemical Industry. (1986). The man–machine interface. *Chemistry and Industry*, (1986), 304–24.

Stefaniak, J. J., Gailey, F. B., Brown, C. S. & Johnson, M. J. (1946). Pilot plant equipment for submerged production of penicillin. *Industrial and Engineering Chemistry*, **38**, 666–71.

Stowell, J. D. & Bateson, J. B. (1983). Economic aspects of industrial fermentations. In *Bioactive Microbial Products 2, Development and Production*, ed. L. J. Nisbet & D. J. Winstanley, pp. 117–39. London: Academic Press.

Vaks, B., Mory, Y., Pederson, J. U. & Horovitz, O. (1984). A semi-continuous process for the production of human interferon-α C from *E. coli*, using tangential-flow microfiltration and immuno-affinity chromatography. *Biotechnology Letters*, **6**, 621–6.

Vandamme, E. J. (ed.) (1984). *Biotechnology of Industrial Antibiotics*. New York: Marcel Dekker.

Vaněk, Z. & Hošťálek, Z. (1973). Molecular basis of polygenic inheritance in the biosynthesis of chlortetracycline. In *Genetics of Industrial Microorganisms*, vol. 2, ed. Z. Vaněk, Z. Hošťálek & J. Cudlin, pp. 353–71. Prague: Academia.

Vaněk, Z. & Hošťálek, Z. (eds.) (1986). *Overproduction of Microbial Metabolites*. Boston, Mass.: Butterworth.

Vass, R. C. & Jefferys, E. G. (1979). Gibberellic acid. In *Secondary Products of Metabolism*, ed. A. H. Rose, pp. 421–33. London: Academic Press.

Villax, I. (1962). *Streptomyces lusitanus* and the problem of classification of the various tetracycline-producing *Streptomyces. Antimicrobial Agents and Chemotherapy*, (1962), 661–8.

Vu-Trong, K. & Gray, P. P. (1982a). Continuous culture studies on the regulation of tylosin biosynthesis. *Biotechnology and Bioengineering*, **24**, 1093–103.

Vu-Trong, K. & Gray, P. P. (1982b). Stimulation of tylosin productivity resulting from cyclic feeding profiles in fed-batch cultures. *Biotechnology Letters*, **4**, 725–8.

Wang, H. Y., Cooney, C. L. & Wang, D. I. C. (1979). Computer control of bakers' yeast production. *Biotechnology and Bioengineering*, **22**, 975–95.

Wegrich, O. G. & Schurter, R. A. Jr (1953). Development of a typical aerobic fermentation. *Industrial and Engineering Chemistry*, **45**, 1153–60.

Weitzman, P. D. J. (1981). Unity and diversity in some bacterial citric acid cycle enzymes. *Advances in Microbial Physiology*, **22**, 185–244.

Williams, S. T., Goodfellow, M., Alderson, G., Wellington, E. M. H., Sneath,

P. H. A. & Sackin, M. J. (1983a). Numerical classification of *Streptomyces* and related genera. *Journal of General Microbiology*, **129**, 1743–813.

Williams, S. T., Goodfellow, M., Wellington, E. M. H., Vickers, J. C., Anderson, G. Sneath, P. H. A., Sackin, M. J. & Mortimer, A. M. A. (1983b). A probability matrix for identification of some streptomycetes. *Journal of General Microbiology*, **129**, 1815–30.

Yamashita, S., Hoshi, H. & Inagaki, T. (1969). Automatic control and optimisation of fermentation processes: glutamic acid. In *Fermentation Advances*, ed. D. Perlman, pp. 441–63. New York: Academic Press.

Young, T. B. & Koplove, H. M. (1972). A systems approach to design and control of antibiotic fermentations. In *Fermentation Technology Today*, ed. G. Terui, pp. 163–6. Osaka: Society of Fermentation Technology, Japan.

Yousefpour, P. & Williams, D. (1981). Real-time optimisation of a fermentation process. *Biotechnology Letters*, **3**, 519–23.

Index

active cells and production, 34
adaptive control, 91
a-factor (Khokhlov), 41
air filters (plant), 162
amino acid syntheses, 53
analytical methods
  cell concentration, 82
  culture volume, 83, 161
  general methods, 82
  product formation, 84
  respiration, 84
anaplerotic pathways, 53
antibiotics
  biosynthesis, 53
  as commercial products, 5
  development steps, 8, 120
  and differentiation, 39–43
  discovery, 5
  and ecology, 6
  screening for, 9, 122
  yield increases, 20 years, 121
anticipatory control, 89
arthrospores and cephalosporin C, 42
assessment of cultures, 93, 195–9

Bacillus subtilis antibiotics, 40
balance in fermentations
  culture and environment, 6, 65, 71
  in fermentation design, 71, 89
  griseofulvin, 69–71
  material balances, 29, 167
  organisms and diverse conditions, 71
  in plant, 200
batch variations, 57–64, 185–99
  early detection, 193
  wrong start, 142, 191
biochemistry of antibiotic fermentations,
  49–56
  ATP, NAD, etc., 50
  biosynthesis of products, 53
  central metabolic system, 52, 53–6
  coenzymes and activation, 50
  effect of fermentation faults, 54
  energy production, 52
  enzyme reactions, 49
  mechanistic cell model, 54
  P/O ratio, 53

  regulation, 50
  respiratory chain, 52
  supplementary routes, 53
  TCA cycle, 52–3
biofactors and differentiation, 41
  in *Achlya bisexualis*, 41
  A-factor (Khokhlov), 41–2
  cytochlasins, 41
biological space, 37
biosynthesis of antibiotics, 53
by-product inhibition
  by cysteine and valine, 125
  by lysine, 53
by-products of fermentations, 37

carbohydrate activation by phosphate, 50
carbohydrate conversion, 52
carbon balance, 29
catabolite repression, 29
  in penicillin, 52, 125
cell behaviour, determinants, 90
cell growth, 21
  colonial growth, 22, 40
  compartmented, 26–8
  curves and phases, 21, 28, 38, 44–5, 47,
    60, 70, 96, 97, 186, 192
  growth models, 31, 66–8, 94–6, 100–3,
    139–42
  growth zones, 27
  particles in growth, 22, 27, 54;
    particle-based model, 22
  pellet formation, 23, 57–62
  submerged, 23
cell measurement (*x*)
  direct, 82
  indirect, 30, 31, 45, 96
cells
  composition, 13
  description, 13
  mechanistic model, 54
  nucleus, 19, 55
  pool, 55
  as production mechanism, 26
  secondary metabolism, 6, 39
  structure and morphology, 12, 23, 47, 55
  walls, eukaryotic and prokaryotic,
    12–14; transport mechanisms, 54